START HERE

A PRACTICAL GUIDE FOR THE OVERWHELMED

DR KERRY MAKIN-BYRD

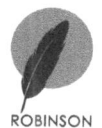

ROBINSON

First published in Great Britain in 2025 by Robinson

10 9 8 7 6 5 4 3 2 1

Copyright © Kerry Makin-Byrd, 2025

Book design by: Catherine Adam, wonderbird.nz
Illustrations by: Katharine Hall, kathallcreative.com

The moral right of the author has been asserted.

Important Note
This book is not intended as a substitute for medical advice or treatment.
Any person with a condition requiring medical attention should consult a qualified medical practitioner or suitable therapist.

All rights reserved.

No part of this publication may be reproduced, stored in a retrieval system, or transmitted, in any form, or by any means, without the prior permission in writing of the publisher, nor be otherwise circulated in any form of binding or cover other than that in which it is published and without a similar condition including this condition being imposed on the subsequent purchaser.

A CIP catalogue record for this book is available from the British Library.

ISBN: 978-1-40878-322-1

Typeset in Mrs Eaves Catherine Adam, wonderbird.nz

Printed and bound in Great Britain by Clays Ltd, Elcograf S.p.A.

Papers used by Robinson are from well-managed forests and other responsible sources.

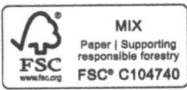

Robinson
An imprint of
Little, Brown Book Group
Carmelite House
50 Victoria Embankment
London EC4Y 0DZ

The authorised representative
in the EEA is
Hachette Ireland
8 Castlecourt Centre
Dublin 15, D15 XTP3, Ireland
(email: info@hbgi.ie)

An Hachette UK Company
www.hachette.co.uk
www.littlebrown.co.uk

Clinical psychologist **Dr Kerry Makin-Byrd** is a noted burnout and wellbeing expert. Alum of Penn State University, University of California, San Francisco and Palo Alto Veterans Affairs Health Care System/Stanford Medical School (affiliated), she was honoured to receive the Special Contribution Award from the Veterans Health Administration in recognition of her impactful policy contributions and clinical teaching. Not only an expert but also a burnout survivor herself, Dr Kerry previously published a memoir, *The Ballad of Burnout*. When she isn't working, Dr Kerry is having fun parenting her daughter, loving her partner of twenty years, and building a mini-mansion for her foster cats.

Praise for *Start Here*

'As a chronically anxious and overwhelmed person, I found in this book a gentle reminder of what is within my control. Kerry helped me reconnect with my own strength, my power and my ability to find peace.'
— **Amie McNee**, author of *We Need Your Art*

'With her latest book, *Start Here*, Dr Makin-Byrd shares a succinct and effective way to meet our stress with kindness and care, offering readers a no-nonsense roadmap for connecting with their deepest intentions.'
— **Sharon Salzberg**, author of *Lovingkindness* and *Real Life*

'This is a rare kind of self-help book – deeply humane, scientifically grounded and courageously honest. Dr Kerry Makin-Byrd brings warmth, clarity and lived wisdom to her three-step model for overcoming overwhelm, one that aligns closely with key psychological flexibility processes. With both rigour and gentleness, she guides the reader towards a life of meaning, compassion and intentional change.'
— **Steven C. Hayes**, Ph.D., Foundation Professor of Psychology Emeritus, University of Nevada, Reno, and originator of Acceptance and Commitment Therapy

'In *Start Here*, Dr Kerry Makin-Byrd offers a refreshingly straightforward roadmap for navigating overwhelm. She guides readers through her simple yet profound framework – soothe, transcend and move – showing how to calm our bodies, widen our perspective and take values-based steps forward. Knowing Kerry personally, I can say that the compassion and clarity you'll find in these pages reflect exactly who she is. This is a book I will be recommending to clients, colleagues and friends alike.'
— **Robyn D. Walser**, PhD, licensed clinical psychologist and author of *The Heart of ACT*, co-author of *You Are Not Your Trauma*, *The Mindful Couple*, *Learning ACT*, *The ACT Workbook for Anger* and *The Moral Injury Workbook*

'It's fitting that I started reading this book in the middle of a personal disaster. What amazed me was how readable it was, even mid-disaster. The first two chapters were breezy and immediately actionable. Despite everything on my to-do list, the steps fit right into my life.

'This book is a breath of fresh air: easy to read, intuitive to apply, and immediately useful. Dr Kerry Makin-Byrd's writing is achingly human. The reality and vulnerability here are rare in a book so compact and clear. That's what makes it powerful – it's both evidence-based and grounded in humanity. Not only was this system created by an expert, it's clearly been used by real humans in difficult situations.

'I love the soothe–transcend–move framework; it's useful for me and my clients. I love how compact and easy to read this book is. Most of all, I love the hope and humanity in every chapter. *Start Here* truly is a "practical guide for the overwhelmed".'

— **Josh Hillis**, author of *Lean and Strong*

'This terrific little book packs a big punch! Dr Kerry distills practical and scientifically based techniques into a simple and digestible format that's perfect for overwhelmed people. You'll finish the book with a clear roadmap for how to soothe yourself, transcend your struggles and change your life for the better. I will be recommending this book to all the overwhelmed people in my life!'

— **Debbie Sorensen**, PhD, clinical psychologist, co-host of *Psychologists Off the Clock*, and author of *ACT for Burnout* and *ACT Daily Journal*

'We all feel overwhelmed at times, and when we do, we can't think clearly enough to find our way out. This book will show you. *Start Here* is like a road map to show you the way towards living well. It's filled with practical strategies, easy-to-read text and fantastic illustrations that form a visual guide. You'll know exactly where to start and be able to follow the three steps towards more energy and recovery. I loved this book, and you will too.'

— **Dr. Louise Hayes**, author of *What Makes You Stronger*, *Your Life, Your Way* and *The Thriving Adolescent*. Developer of DNA-V, clinical psychologist and adjunct senior research fellow at La Trobe University, Melbourne

'Kerry Makin-Byrd is one of the most insightful and wise psychologists I know, and she has shared her whole heart and wisdom in *Start Here*. This is a book you'll reach for time and time again as life throws you new challenges; each time a different exercise or heart-felt sentence will hit the spot for you.'

— **Ben Sedley**, author of *Holding the Heavy Stuff*

To my clients

Thank you for trusting me

Thank you for teaching me

Contents

The ending	01
1. How to address overwhelm, prevent burnout and save your life	03
2. Soothe	09
3. Transcend	25
4. Move	51
5. End here and keep going	71
Appendix: Dr Kerry's annual review	89
Acknowledgements	98
Endnotes	100
Behaviour change form references	109

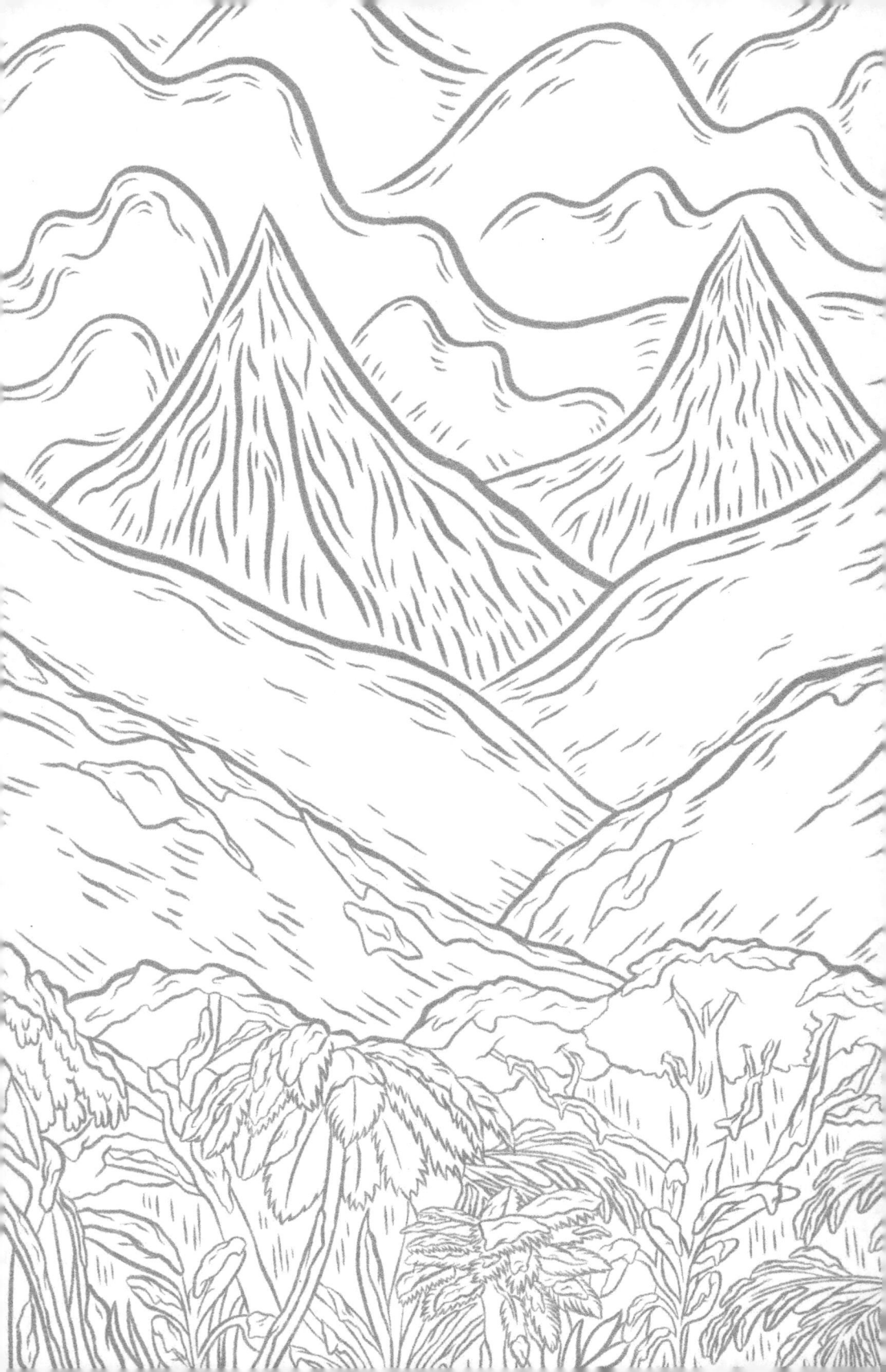

The Ending

Here is the ending, placed at the beginning.
Overcoming overwhelm requires three steps:

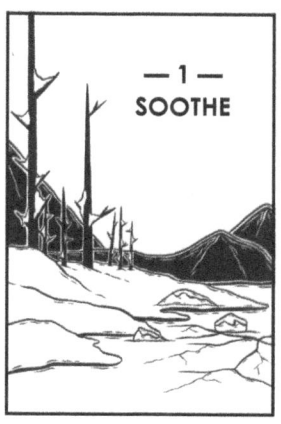
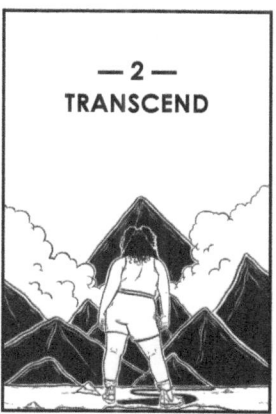
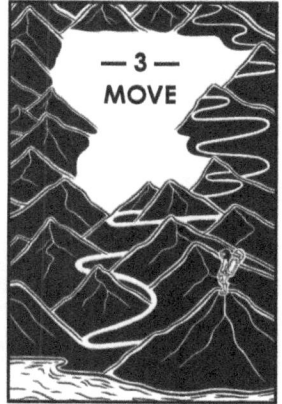

After a little practice, you can complete these three steps in less than a minute. For example:

» Notice that you are overwhelmed *(three seconds)*.

» **Soothe:** Take a long, slow breath *(seven seconds)*.

» **Transcend:** Name your thoughts, emotions and physical sensations *(eighteen seconds)*.

» **Move:** Remind yourself of your defining value or goal for this moment and take the first small action towards that goal *(twenty seconds)*.

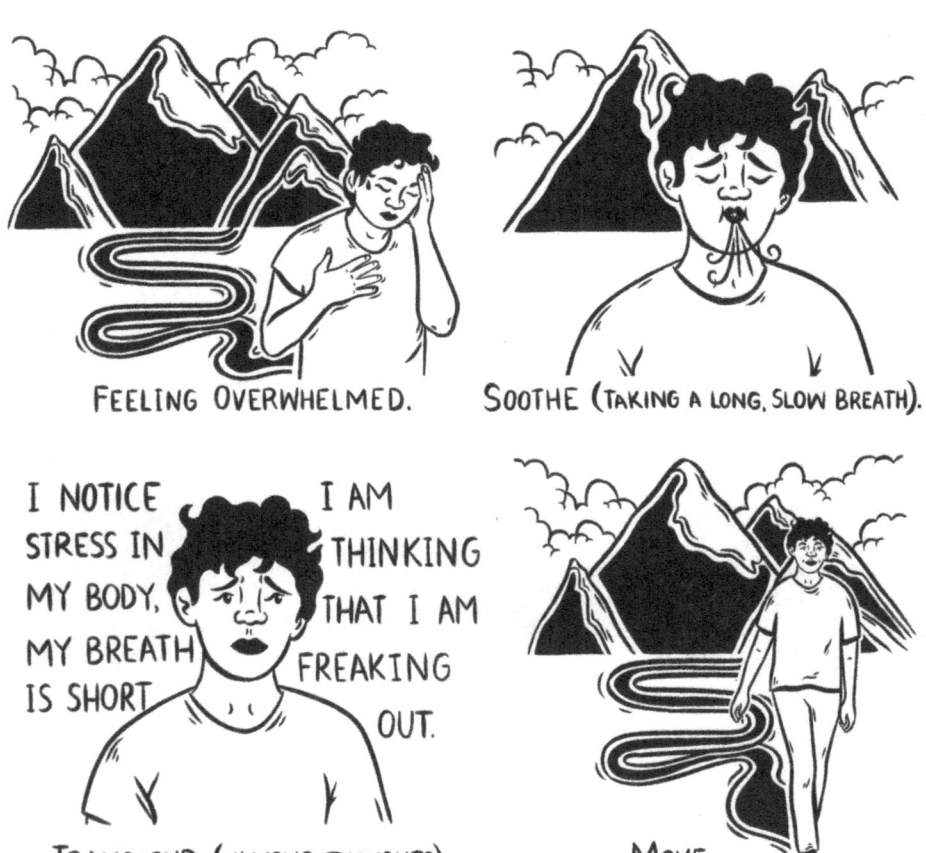

With practice, you can pause, breathe, list your sensations and thoughts and move forward in less than one minute.

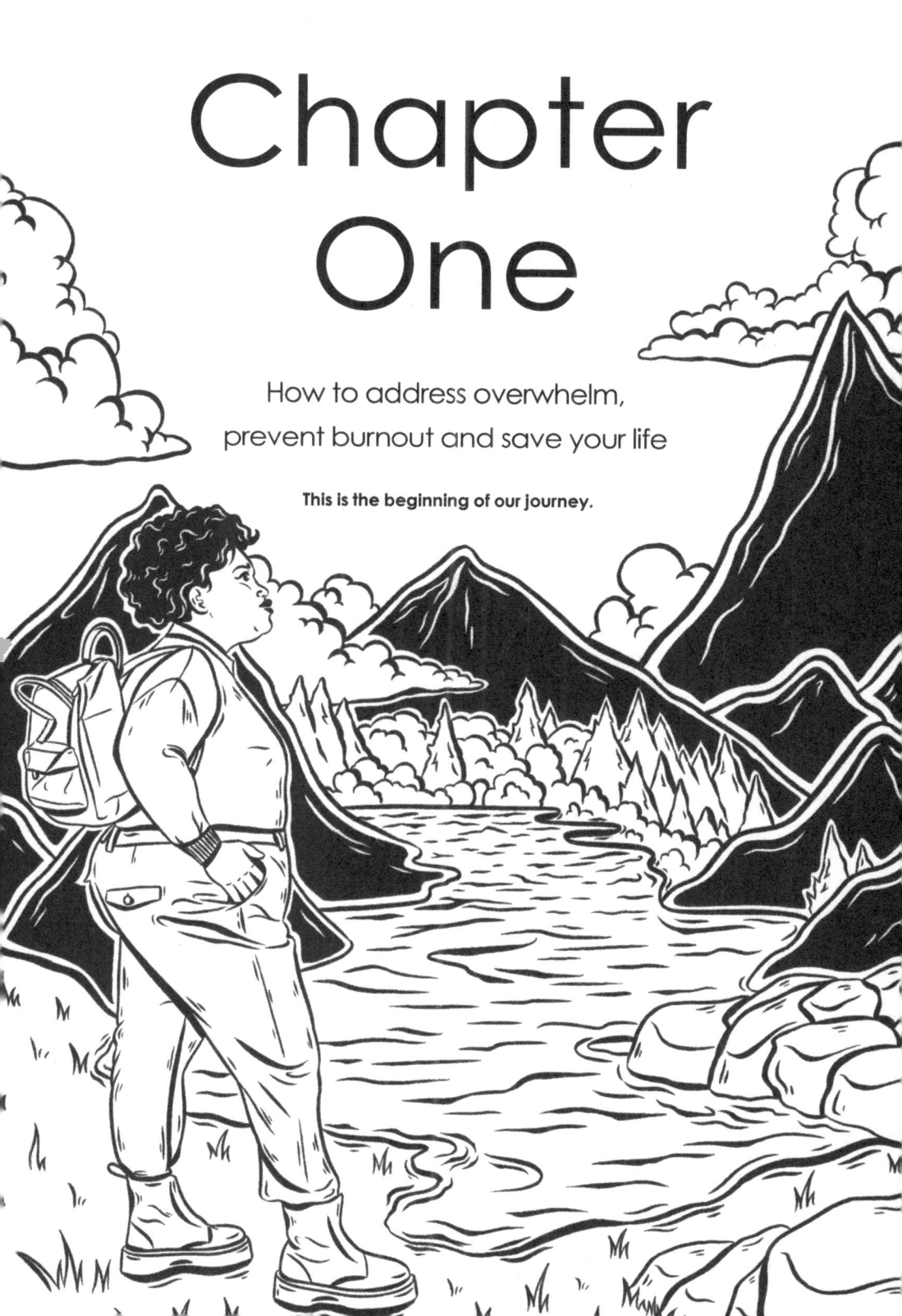

I woke up with my heart pounding in my chest. Again.

Breathing in short gasps, I replayed the worst moments of the last few days: my cousin's escalating anxiety symptoms, the overwhelm and minutiae of planning a six-day camping trip, an argument with a friend. Not large traumas, just the normal moments of life, piled high and deep, layering over me. Like waves crashing over my head, I was desperate for time or space to catch a breath. Each day this week I was tighter, less focused and quicker to anger. Each night I had less sleep, startling awake from a nightmare at 2, 3 or 4 a.m.

I'm a clinical psychologist. Each day I teach people the tools of self-soothing, gaining perspective and moving forward from overwhelm. But tonight, all those tools were inaccessible.

I scrolled desperately through my phone . . . eight meditation apps and I still felt lost.

'I need a manual!' I thought.

I wanted a guide to tell me in clear, simple language how to walk myself out of overwhelm, step by step. I needed how-to instructions so that I could pick myself out of the crashing surf and sit back on the rocky shore.

This is that manual. There are three key steps: soothe, transcend and move.

We will learn tools to soothe ourselves when we're stuck in a fight-or-flight response.

Then, we will learn to transcend a difficult moment, widening and realigning our perspective.

Finally, as we are enjoying our calmer and more spacious stance, we will ground ourselves in our values and make a plan for moving forward.

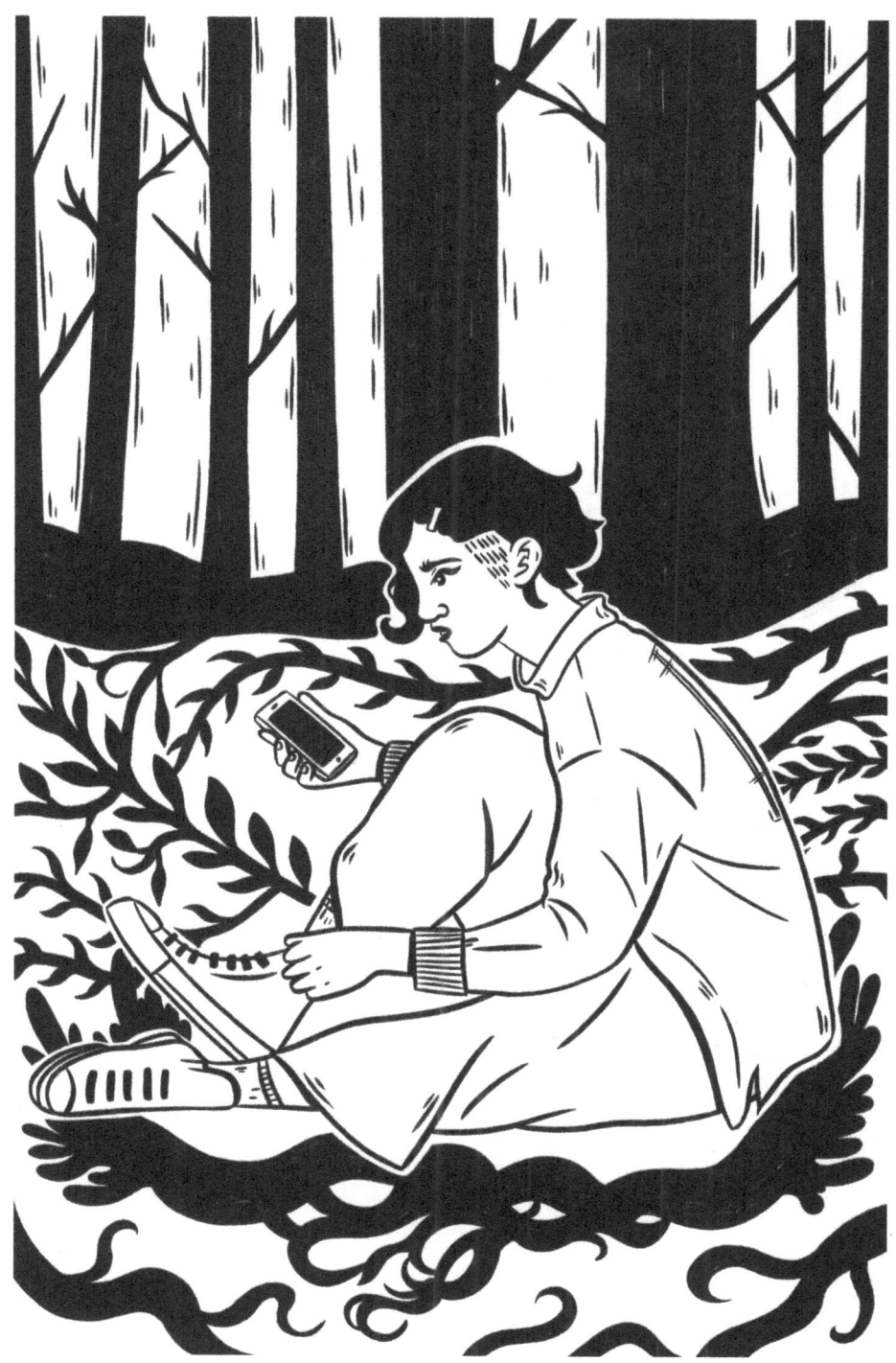

I was stuck in overwhelm with eight meditation apps and no peace.

This book is a compendium of advice. It is built of bits of science-backed learning that helped me, hundreds of my clients and thousands of research participants. I hope it may help you. But before we get into all the details of how to apply the three steps to your life, I want to give a warning.

The fields of psychology, psychiatry and medicine were built mainly by white men of European descent.[i,ii] The tools I suggest below are still not widely replicated across age, caste[iii] or cultural background.[iv,v] For too long, clinical psychology has heavily favoured individual self-help while under-emphasising the wide, large influence of community- and system-level factors.[vi]

> This book is deeply imperfect.
> It is limited by my own vantage point
> and the limited science.[vii]

Given these limitations, only you can decide whether these words are helpful or harmful tools for your own growth. Our science is still so limited. You deserve more and better. But more and better science isn't here today. This is what we have, and this is what I can offer, humbly and with warning.

Trust your experience, your heart and your senses.

Let's go gently, taking what is useful and discarding the rest.

Long story short, handle with care.
Hold these lessons with care.
Hold yourself with care.

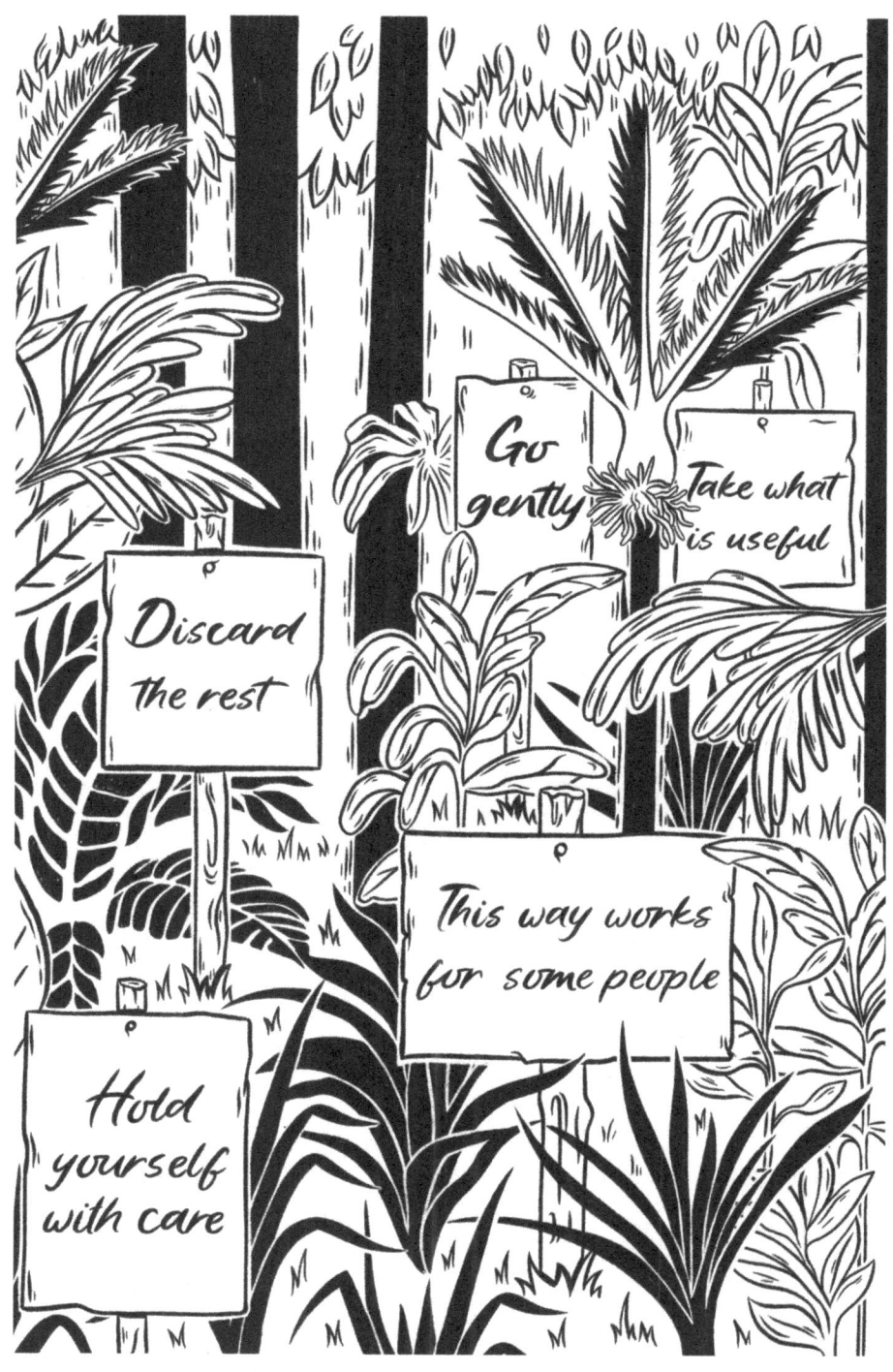

Our tools of guidance are still not widely replicated.

Each chapter of this book uses the same format. We begin by doing. Each skill, tool and practice comes with clear, brief instructions. After a practical recipe for how to do the step, there is a fuller description of the data and science rationale, or the how and why, tucked after the skill instructions for those who are interested.

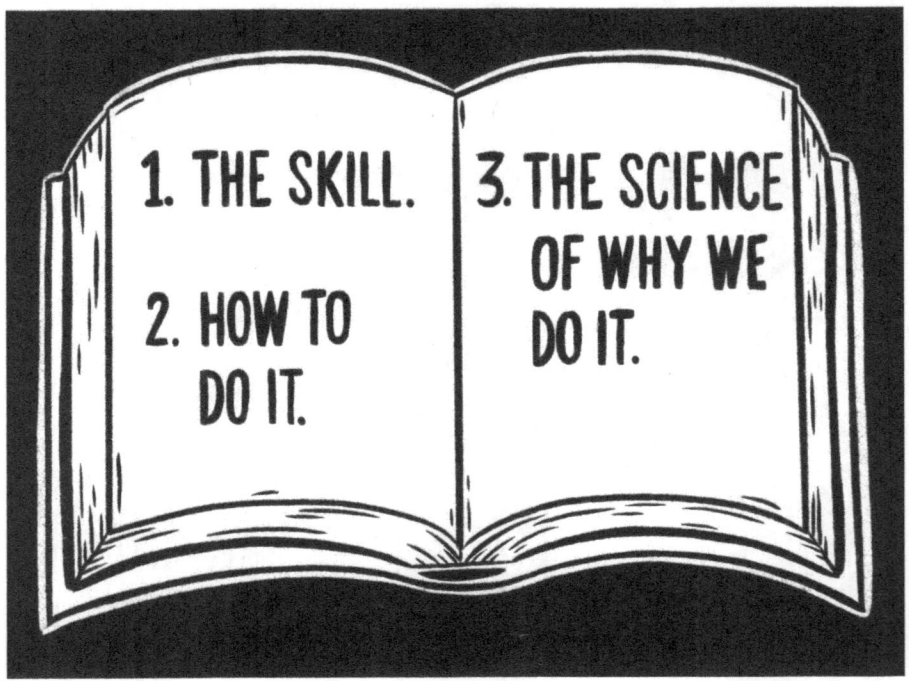

Each chapter of this book uses the same format.

No matter where you are and what is happening in your life, there are concrete evidence-backed tools that can help. Practise a few simple exercises and you can:

» **soothe** yourself back to a calmer mindset
» **transcend** the minor and major crises of the day
» and **move** forward with hope and clarity.

Yes, that sounds like a lot.

It starts with just one step.

Let's start together.

Chapter Two

Soothe

Imagine we arrive at a frozen lake at the base of a mountain.

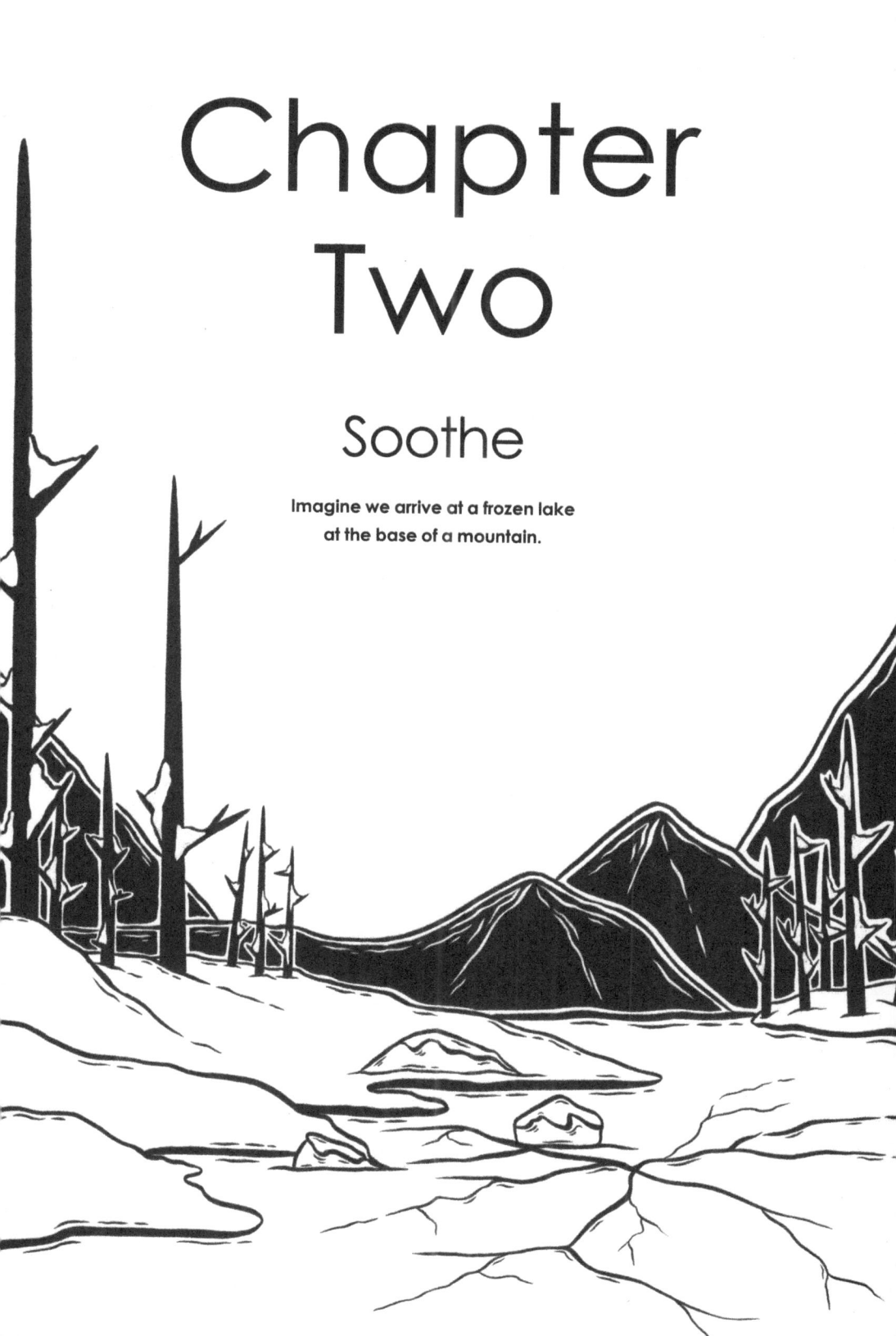

What we're doing

When stressed and overwhelmed, our body activates its threat system.[1] Our threat system was designed via evolution to keep us safe. It was intended to physiologically prepare us for situations like fighting a bear, fleeing a snake or freezing as a woolly mammoth lumbered by. Now, this threat system is sometimes triggered by a variety of stressful (but non-fatal) scenarios in our day-to-day lives.

When we read the news about distant tragedies, receive a bill that is overdue for payment, or lead an online meeting, our threat system can be activated. We may react as though we are in physical danger, experiencing classic cues of the fight-or-flight response such as a pounding heart, rushes of adrenaline and a defensive stance. In this activated state, we become myopic, focused only on the perceived danger in front of us. This is a useful tool when a bear walks towards us, less helpful when the threat is a pile of small demands that we feel unable to prioritise. Sometimes the stress is so large or constant that we experience freeze, characterised by immobilisation, numbness and physical shutdown.

When we are panicked under physically safe conditions, our first step is to soothe ourselves. We must calm our bodies. When our mind, heart and body know that we are safe, our frontal lobe (which is the most recently evolved part of our brain and an expert on perspective-taking) is welcomed back to the planning party.

Note, I am offering a tasting platter of practices in the following pages. There are many options; pick one or two that work for you then practise them frequently. McKay[ii] suggests 'two or three daily practice sessions for at least a week' to gain mastery.

With regular practice you will notice that you start to automatically soothe yourself as your body becomes tense. This is a subtle but powerful shift. You are practising and practising, then one day you notice yourself taking a long, deep breath, stretching your neck or rolling your shoulders as stress enters, not after it has tied you in knots.

> Slowly, slowly, this change begins
> with what you do today.

Practice 1: Chill out

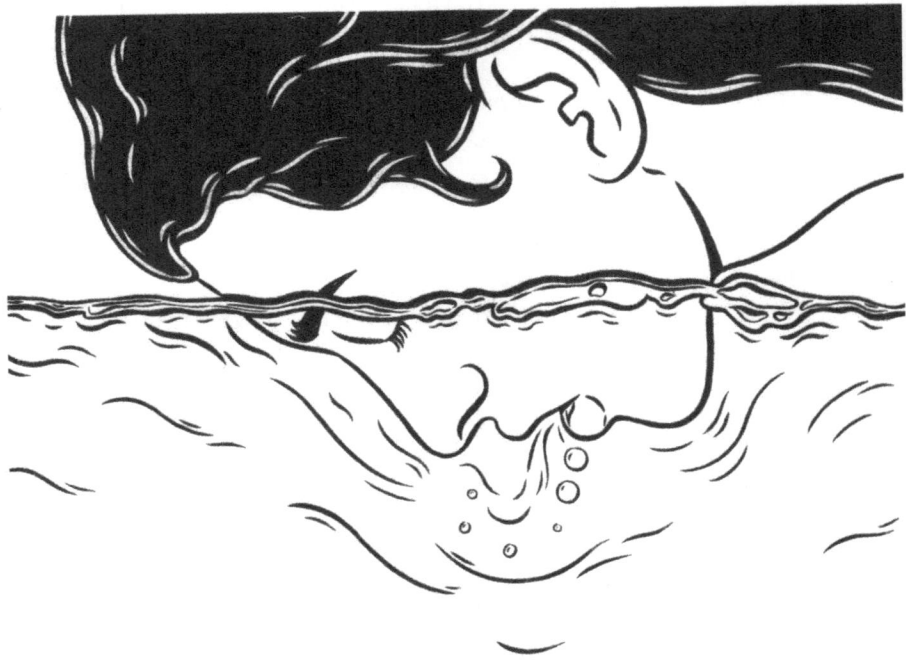

Submerge your face in cold water to induce the calming diving reflex.

Quickly calm your heart rate and breathing by holding your breath and submerging your face in cold water for about thirty seconds. Feel free to do this multiple times. Don't want to dunk your face in cold water? (Yep, welcome to the club. Literally no one likes doing this at first.)

Here are some milder options:

» Place a cold cloth or ice pack on the back, right side of your neck.

» Take a cold shower or, even better, a cold bath.[iii]

» Put an ice pack or packet of frozen peas on your forehead and eyes.

A few years ago, my family and I camped in the mountains 4,100 metres above sea level. It was beautiful, our tent nestled among a circle of friends' tents tucked below blazing stars.

The first night, I couldn't sleep. All I could focus on was my daughter's laboured breathing. Her typically mild asthma had flared as we hiked during the day. I listened to the pitched whistle as her lungs worked for air. In a backdrop of soft forest noises, as owls called across the trees and the wind nudged breezes, I could feel my own panicked brain rapidly flipping through the problems: no phone service, at least an hour from the nearest medical centre, one pathetic little steroid inhaler. My heart raced, my own breathing short and shallow, escalating till I couldn't hear anything over a roar of panic in my ears. This was the first time I truly needed my own 'chill out'.

The reality was my daughter was all right. She was breathing, consistently and softly. We had medicine and could get her to medical care if we needed it. But I couldn't see any of that.

In a small burst of clarity among the haze of my panic, I heard the bubbling creek next to our tent. I slipped out of the sleeping bag, unzipped the tent flap as quietly as possible, and with my breath still coming in short bursts, crawled over to the stream.

I teach this skill all the time, and the visions of all my clients who have used it urged me on. I dunked my head in the stream, snowmelt flowing over my hair and down my face. I gasped at the icy shock.

An ancient mechanism took the controls. My ears opened, my head cleared and my breathing returned to long, slow cycles.

🔍 DATA

When we immerse our face in cold water or apply a cold cloth to the back, right section of our neck[iv] we induce the diving reflex.[v] The diving reflex is a handy term for a range of calming physiological changes that occur in our bodies when presented with cold water. Blood is diverted to your brain and heart, your vessels constrict and your spleen contracts.[vi,vii] In studies, people who submerge their face in cold water experience lower heart rates, and lower anxiety and panic symptoms post-dip.[viii] After applying a cold face mask, people experience better recovery from continued stressors, and lower cortisol response to ongoing stress.[ix] Yes, dipping your face in icy water sounds cold and cringy, but it can be a useful first step to soothing ourselves.

Practice 2: Breathe

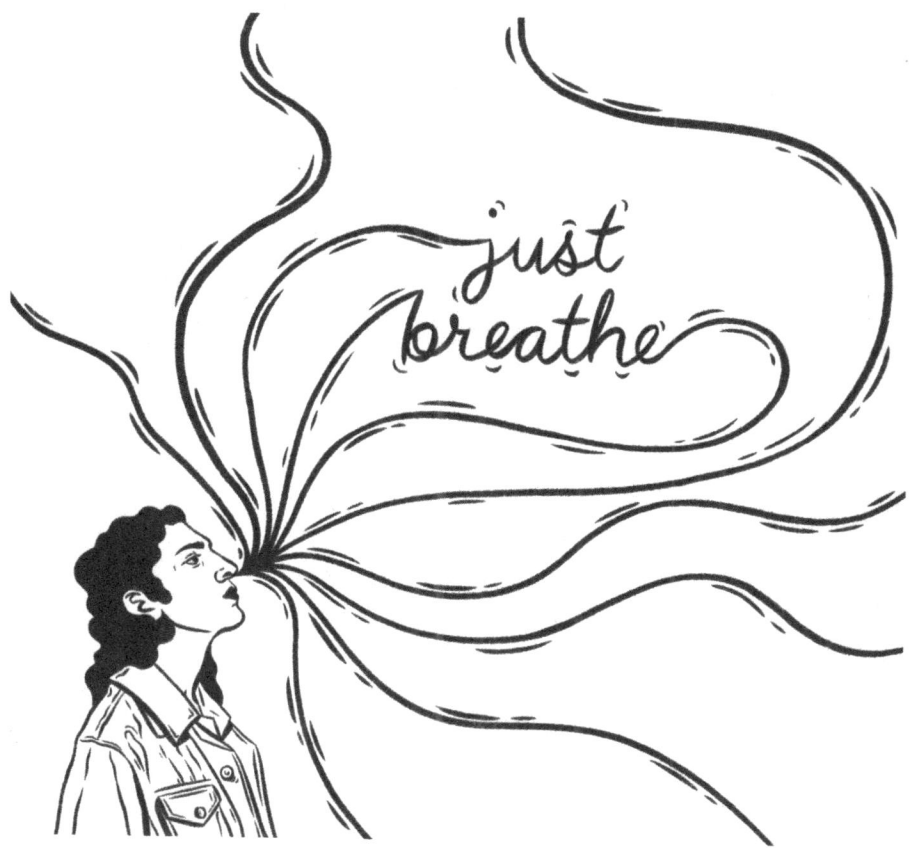

Just breathe. The advice is so common it's cliché. And yet, breath is always available to us, with no special tools required.

Option 2a: Long exhale breathing

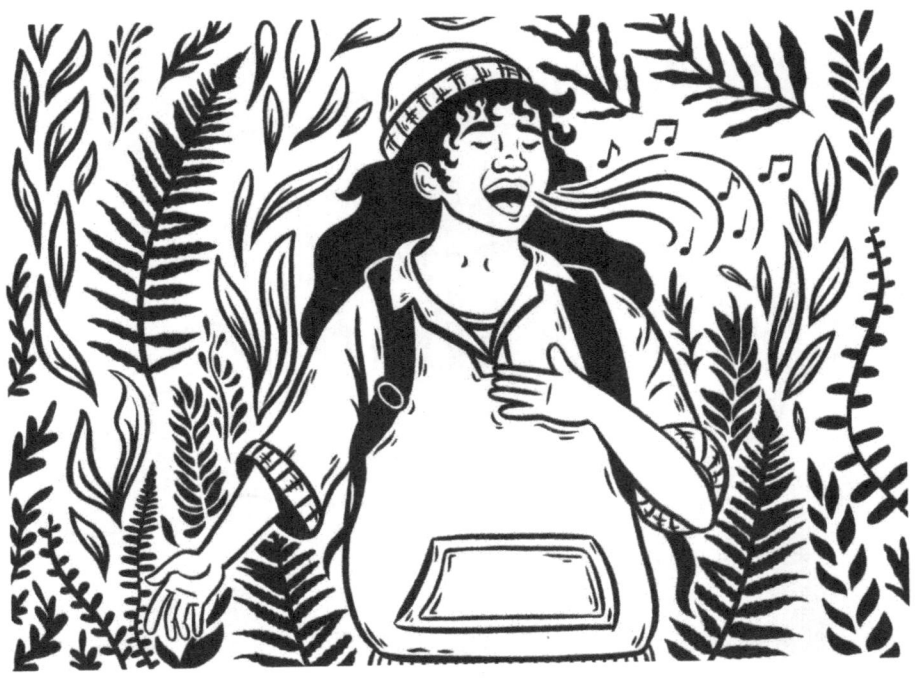

Soothe yourself by breathing or singing with extended exhales.

» For five to ten minutes, just sit quietly and breathe. Focus on inhaling through your nose and then slowly exhaling through your mouth.

» During this time, your mind can:

1. count your breaths from one to ten (then restart at one), or

2. label the breath as it occurs, 'in . . . out . . . in . . . out' or 'inhale . . . exhale . . . inhale . . . exhale', or

3. focus on the prominent physical sensations when breathing, such as the movement of your torso or the movement of air on your top lip.

Singing a long comforting song to yourself can also work! Because when you're enjoying your favourite Adele hit, you're inhaling then doing a longggggg exhale to belt out that ballad. Voilà!

Option 2b: Diaphragmatic breathing

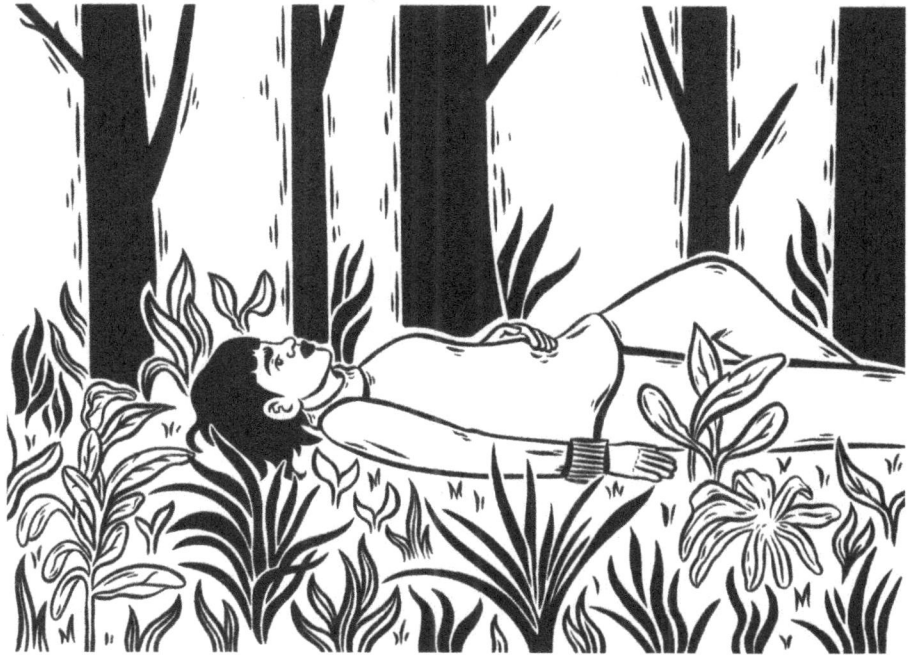

Inhaling, imagining we are filling our lower back with nourishing air.

With diaphragmatic breathing, we focus on long, deep inhales that fill our diaphragm, which lives down below your lungs. Practise any of the options below for five to ten minutes a day.

» **Seated:** Place one hand on your chest, the other just above your belly button. Inhale deeply, so the hand on your belly moves and your chest remains still.

» **Lying down:** Lie on your back, placing an object on your stomach. Focus on inhaling to lift the object (like a stuffed toy), then on deep, long exhaling.

» **Adaptation:** Lie face down, focusing on your abdominal muscles pressing into the ground as you inhale.

🔍 DATA

Breathing practices have been used in contemplative and medical traditions for centuries, to calm the body and strengthen focus.[x] The unique power of breathing with a prolonged exhale[xi] (or 'low inhale to exhale ratio' breathing) was initially demonstrated in the 1980s.[xii]

Multiple studies have suggested that diaphragmatic breathing can lead to decreased psychological and physiological stress.[xiii] Deep and slow breathing raises pain thresholds and reduces feelings of tension and anger.[xiv]

Even five minutes of long exhale breathing a day significantly increases people's mood and slows their breathing rate across a month of practice.[xv]

Practice 3: Body relaxation

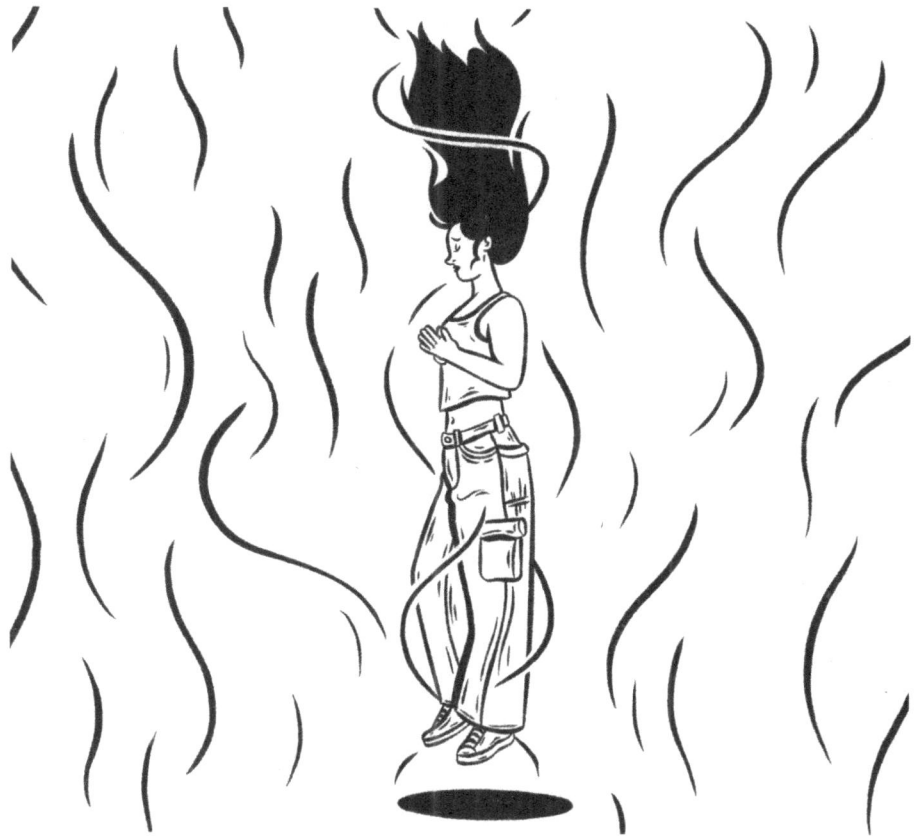

We can also soothe ourselves by focusing on our bodies.

Breathing exercises aren't for everyone, especially people prone to hyperventilation or panic. Full body relaxation can be a powerful alternative.

Option 3a: Progressive muscle relaxation

This exercise takes about twenty minutes. For each muscle group, you will:

- » tense the specific muscle group for five seconds[xvi]
- » fully release the muscle group for ten seconds, savouring the sensations of relaxation
- » then take three long, deep breaths.

Tense and release each muscle group in the following order:

1. right hand and lower arm
2. left hand and lower arm
3. right upper arm
4. left upper arm
5. forehead
6. face
7. jaw
8. neck
9. chest, shoulders and upper back
10. abdomen
11. right thigh
12. left thigh
13. right calf, toe pointed down
14. left calf, toe pointed down
15. right calf, toe pointed up
16. left calf, toe pointed up.

Option 3b: Autogenics

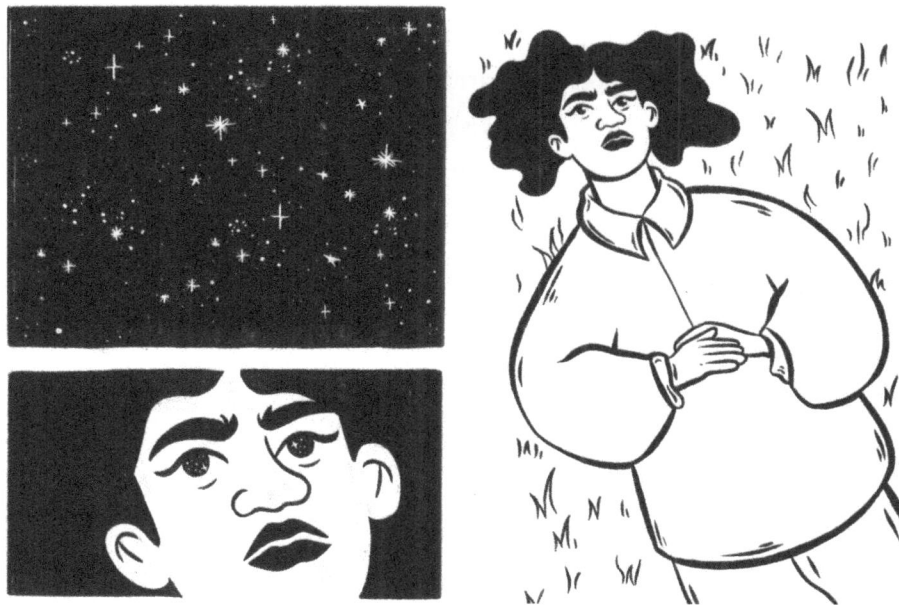

Imagine you are lying under a big night sky.

Autogenic training is a relaxation technique that soothes the autonomic nervous system via a series of statements about the warmth and heaviness of the body. You can use a similar script each day, building from 'heavy' to 'warm' to 'heavy and warm', and so on. (This might seem confusing, but I promise it's not – just follow the full script on the next page.)

» Find a quiet, private place to practise.

» Sit or lie down, closing your eyes or just softening your gaze.

» As you read the script,[xvii] settle your attention on the area of your body as you refer to it.

» Be curious and non-judgemental, just noticing the sensations in the body part.

Aloud or in your mind, repeat the following:

Heavy
    My right arm is heavy
    My left arm is heavy
    Both of my arms are heavy
    My right leg is heavy
    My left leg is heavy
    Both of my legs are heavy
    My arms and legs are heavy

Warm
    My right arm is warm
    My left arm is warm
    Both of my arms are warm
    My right leg is warm
    My left leg is warm
    Both of my legs are warm
    My arms and legs are warm

Heavy and Warm
    My right arm is heavy and warm
    My left arm is heavy and warm
    Both of my arms are heavy and warm
    My right leg is heavy and warm
    My left leg is heavy and warm
    Both of my legs are heavy and warm
    My arms and legs are heavy and warm
    My breath is slow and steady
    My heartbeat is calm and regular

Together
    My arms are heavy and warm
    My legs are heavy and warm
    My breath is slow and steady
    My heartbeat is calm and regular
    My middle is warm
    My forehead is cool

🔍 DATA

Medical professionals have been prescribing body-based relaxation skills for almost a century. Autogenic training was first described in 1959.[xviii] Even earlier, progressive muscle relaxation was popularised in the bluntly, bemusingly titled 1934 book, *You Must Relax*.[xix] These skills have been used in stress management, health and psychology interventions for decades.[xx]

Body relaxation skills lead to reductions in self-reported stress, as well as lowered cortisol markers, commonly considered physiological evidence of stress.[xxi] While most studies evaluate programmes that are weeks long,[xxii] happily there is also evidence that **even a single session can be useful**. Hundreds of college students reported lower anxiety after only a twenty-minute body relaxation practice, and when exposed to stress later, the people who learned the body relaxation skill recovered more quickly compared to people who were not taught the skill.[xxiii]

Wrap-up

When life seems to be swirling around you, when you feel tied tight, nauseous, fractious or weepy, soothe yourself first. Calm the body and quiet the threat response.

- » You can use the diving reflex, quieting your heart and respiration, enjoying the same benefits as if plunging into cool, deep water.
- » You can use long exhale breathing, placing one hand on your heart and one on your belly to notice the movement of your lower torso while keeping your chest still.
- » Or use guided visualisation to imagine that your body is warm and heavy, starting with your arms, then legs, then breath and heartbeat.

Any of these tools will ready us for the next step: accessing more recently evolved parts of our brain to gain perspective.

Chapter Three

Transcend

Next, we climb higher, to gain new perspective on what is leading to overwhelm.

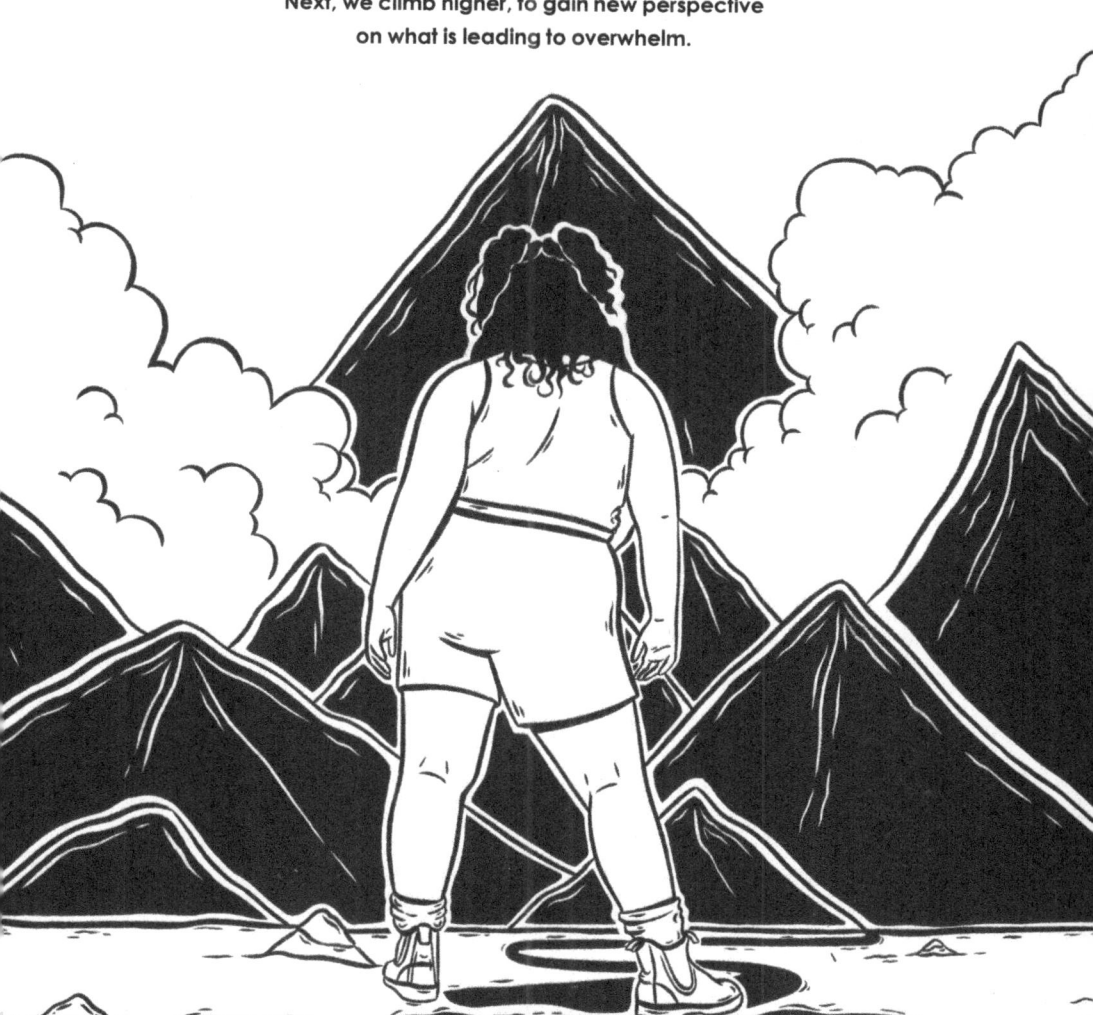

I've had two bouts of professional burnout (so far). With each round, I dug myself into a hole of work obsession where everything else in my life faded into the background. I ignored friends, then lost them. I either exercised obsessively, assuming that would fix everything, or ignored my body entirely, till my new normal was a chronic, dull headache and a body so exhausted I fell asleep every time I sat down.

Anaïs Nin reminds us that blossoming comes only when changing is less painful than remaining in our stagnant sameness. Happily for me, at some point, burnout hurt more than changing. I hurt enough that I was willing to consider giving up my old ways, my faster/better/more tools of self-destruction.

Addicts call this rock bottom. At this wonderful rock bottom, I could begin to transcend the details keeping me stuck. At my low point, I was willing to look at reality just as it was.

I was finally able to see my unsustainable job and my insufficient resources and balancing skills. Then, I began to practise self-kindness, gradually learning to be as sweet to my own exhausted self as I would be to any other helper plagued by vicarious trauma. After clear seeing and self-compassion, I was ready to be flexible, to see my situation from many perspectives, and to begin to find a way out.

Now you will learn these same skills.

What we're doing

Now that your breath and heartbeat are slow and steady, it is time to examine what is causing the overwhelm in your life. Transcending the details that keep us stuck begins by courageously looking at what is. When we are soothed, we can begin to filter out our dreams of what we yearn to be true and the fears that chase us away from clear seeing.

Seeing reality as it is right now is simple for me to suggest but harder for all of us to apply in our lives. And, like any skill, we can get better with practice, especially as we learn more about our common filters and blind spots. As we get stronger at viewing things as they are, instead of how we wish them to be, then we can evaluate what isn't working. Finally, we figure out how to change what we can and accept what we can't.

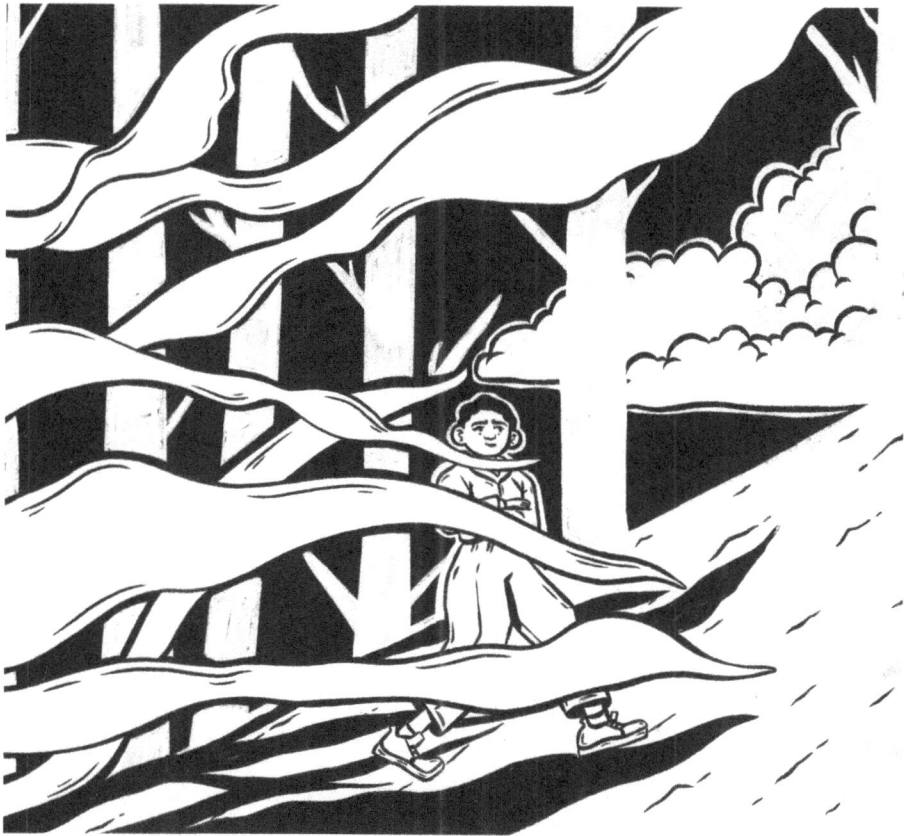

We must practise seeing things as they are instead of how we wish them to be.

Practice 1: Clear seeing

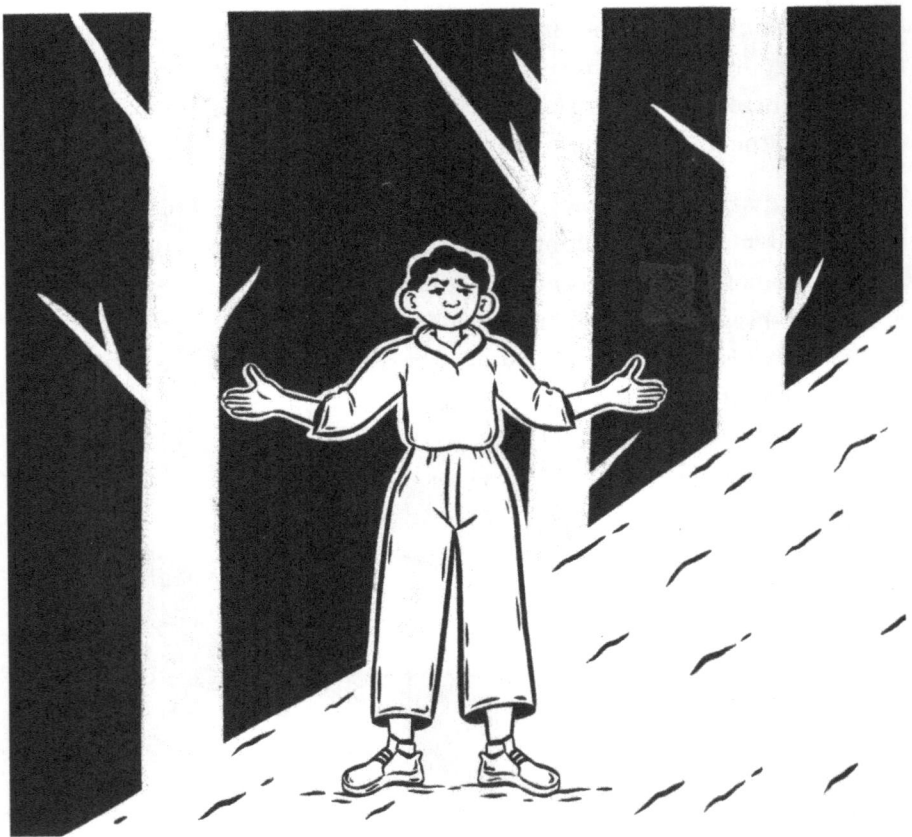

When we begin by acknowledging *this is what is*, we stop arguing with realities that we can't change.

Our (next) first step is to look bravely at what is happening. We decided to do something about our overwhelm. We decided to dip our heads in cold water, breathe deeply and say, 'no more'.

Here we go.

I stopped using the word 'acceptance' in my clinical work because when many people hear acceptance, they translate it to mean submission or a stamp of approval.

Understandably, people don't want to say, *yes please, OK by me*, to the things that keep them up at night. So instead of acceptance, I suggest the term 'clear seeing'. When we begin by acknowledging *this is what is*, we stop arguing with realities that we can't change. It isn't easy, but it is important. When we stop the useless fighting, we have more attention and intention to construct *what will be*. Let's soothe ourselves as we need to, then take a steely-eyed view of what is causing our overwhelm.

Option 1a: Write out the problem

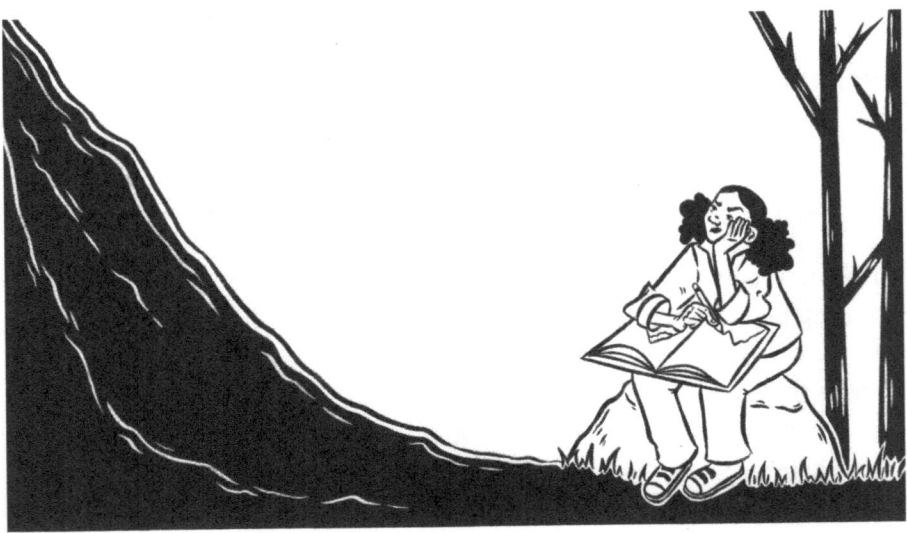

When we write or draw, we naturally create distance and perspective from our problems.

Imagine you are writing a letter to a loved one – really lay out all your thoughts and emotions. (Sometimes people feel worried that if they start opening up, they'll never stop. I promise you, in fifteen years of emotional conversations, this has never happened.)

1. List all the things that are overwhelming you right now.
2. What are the parts that you don't have control over? (For example, how someone else is behaving, what someone else wants, how X will turn out, etc.)
3. Of all the things that you can't control, which drives you the most crazy? (These are the places we're really arguing with reality.)
4. What would you have to feel or experience if you accepted that you can't control these parts? What would it mean? What would then be true? (Ugh, yes, this part can be tough.)
5. Now what are the parts of the problem that you can control? (Hint: this is typically simply your own behaviour.)
6. To review: I am feeling overwhelmed by _____. I really want to control _____, but I know I can't. I can only control _____.

Option 1b: Explain the problem

This is a list of questions you can talk through with a friend. Bonus hint: this works just as well if you send your friend a long video or audio memo answering these questions. Even walking through the forest having an imaginary conversation with your loved one can work the same transcending magic.

1. Describe all the problems you're struggling with. Really get into the details, with a special focus on how you're feeling, what thoughts you're having and where you feel stuck.
2. In your heart of hearts, are you absolutely stuck? Or, deep down, do you have a teeny sense of what might help or where you could go from here?
3. Then:
    a. If you are absolutely stuck, what information or support do you need to learn more or get moving?
    b. If you suspect that you might prefer staying stuck, what is the hard truth that you don't want to see,
    or know,
    or do?
    (Dude, welcome to the club, we have *all* been here.)
4. Now speak for your friend. What would they say? Where do they agree and empathise? What is their advice?

Option 1c: Rain

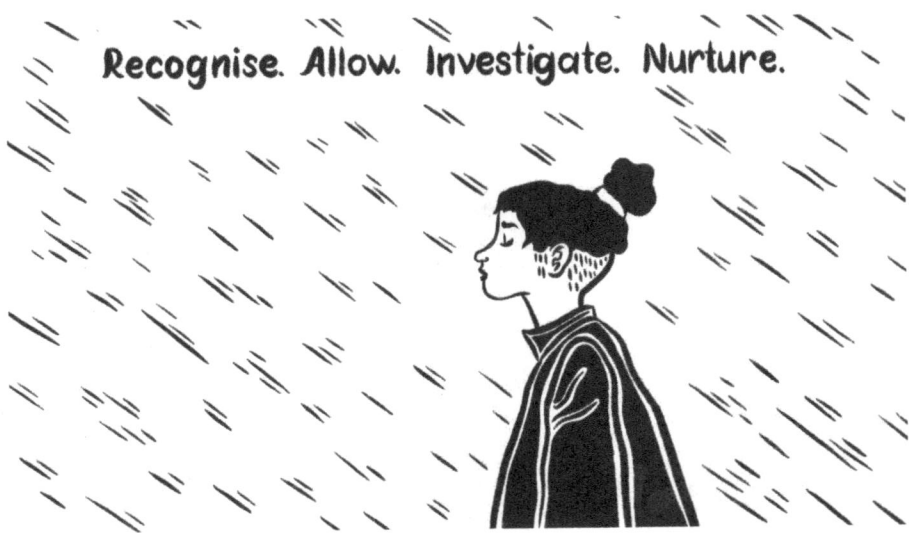

Gentle as warm, soft rain on your face, this simple acronym is a useful guide.

Developed by Michelle McDonald[i] and popularised by Tara Brach,[ii] you can use the RAIN (Recognise | Allow | Investigate | Nurture) acronym to examine your experience with warmth and curiosity.

» **R**ecognise that this is difficult. Breathe slowly, noticing your thoughts, emotions, physical sensations and urges.

» **A**llow the experiences to be there, just as they are. Imagine that you are a wide, deep ocean; each sensation is simply a wave.

» **I**nvestigate the layers of experience with curiosity and kindness. Breathe into the tense parts. This is especially helpful if you notice something distracting, painful or sticky.

» **N**urture or nourish the parts that are hard or tight. Breathe deeply, with a long exhale. Imagine that, with each breath, you are relaxing and opening, sending love to difficult places.

Practise a grounding mantra such as 'this is what is';
'this is a wave . . . I am the ocean', or 'I am here, I am safe'.

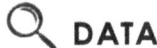 **DATA**

Acceptance has been taught within religious and contemplative traditions for centuries. In recent times, the fields of psychology and medicine have shown that we can reduce our physical pain[iii] and psychological suffering by building psychological acceptance. Mindfulness interventions[iv] teach learners to practise a non-judgemental, warm and curious stance to look at *what is*. Without diving into formal meditation practices, we are cultivating acceptance and openness in the brief exercises above.

We can reduce our struggles when we struggle against reality less.

Hayes and colleagues describe this practice as taking an 'open, receptive, flexible and nonjudgemental posture'[v] to our experiences. Across a wide variety of third-wave cognitive and behavioural therapies,[vi] the specific exercises may look different, but the overarching goals are the same: to build psychological acceptance and openness while decreasing avoidance and rigidity.

As you completed any of the clear-seeing exercises above, you were practising openness and acceptance. You were undermining your avoidance, instead being warm and curious about what is keeping you stuck.

Practice 2: Self-compassion

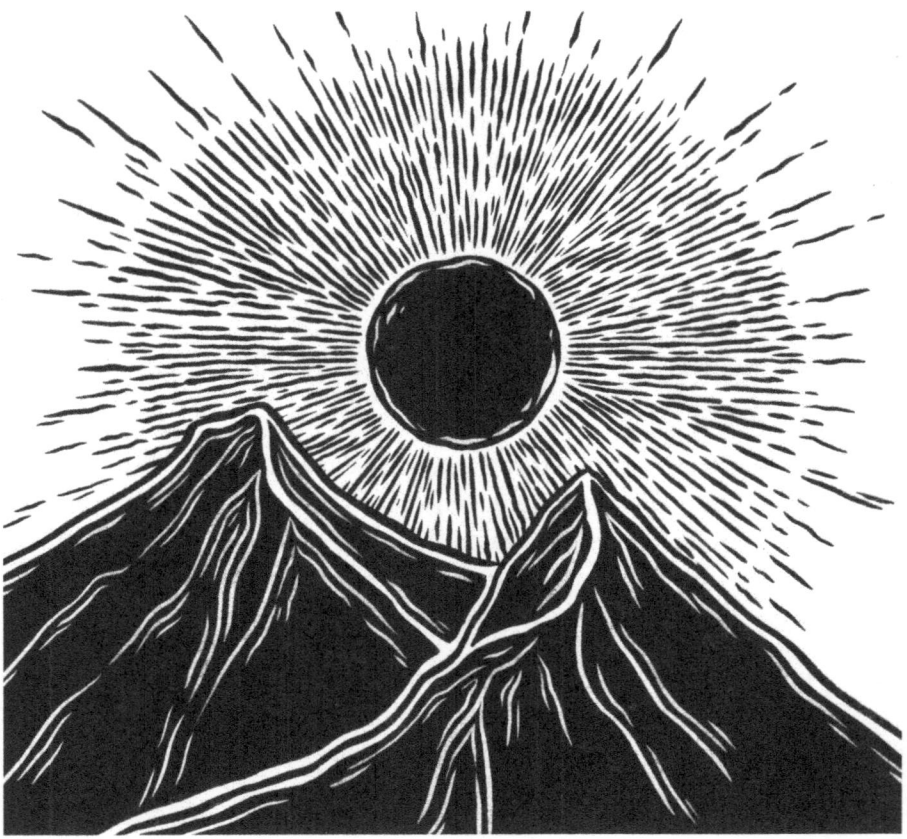

Imagine you are receiving love from a force larger than yourself, like a steady, warm sun.

Some people find that after clear-seeing, they are ready to jump ahead to Practice 3: Perspective-taking/metacognition, or even to move to the next chapter to start planning changes. If that's not you, no problem, keep reading. Self-compassion is here to help.

Some people are scared of learning or practising self-compassion. You may be worried you won't know how to be kind to yourself or that you will be overwhelmed by emotions.

Some people fear that if they are kinder to themselves, they will:

» become weak

» lose their edge, or

» be self-compassionate even when they don't 'deserve' it.

These fears are normal . . . and unhelpful (they are also inaccurate; more on this later).

Worries about being soft get in the way of adding one more skill to your tool belt. Self-compassion, as defined by Dr Kristin Neff, comprises three facets: (a) awareness of your emotional pain; (b) recognition that all people experience these feelings (i.e. our sadness, guilt or upset is a common experience of being human); and (c) a balanced, proportional view of the pain.[vii]

When we are self-compassionate, we acknowledge something feels hard, without avoiding or collapsing into the darkest depths. On pages 36–39 I've listed three of my favourite ways to practise self-compassion. Experiment with each one and see what works best for you!

Option 2a: The self-compassionate letter

Oh, the power of writing yourself a letter.[viii] Nothing calls us to be so honest and direct as the prospect of having a private word with ourselves about this beautiful mess we are in. Get settled in a quiet room with a pen and paper.

- Begin the standard way: Dear Kerry . . .
- Step 1: **Mindfulness**. Begin by remembering a recent difficult situation or stressor. This should be a six out of ten, not the most overwhelming or traumatic experience you have had.
- Write about the situation, focusing not on the details of what happened but instead on how you felt – your thoughts, feelings, what you were yearning for and needing.
- Write about both the stress/suffering and the core need underneath it. For example, the desire for health, safety, love, appreciation, connection or achievement.
- Step 2: **Common humanity**. This experience, your experience, is common to all humanity. Provide empathy and validation. Many people in this situation would feel just like you. Everyone has experienced this or something similar. We all make mistakes or get angry or feel lonely. This isn't because there's something wrong with you (or me); it is just the reality of being human.
- Step 3: **Mentor** yourself with some compassionate advice or encouragement. What would you say to a loved one in this situation? What would you say to someone who you believed in wholeheartedly and wanted the best for?

Ahh. Big sigh. You did it. Take a minute to reread it, silently or aloud. Notice how it feels. Now tuck it away for the next time you need a boost of self-kindness and perspective.

Example:

Dear Kerry,

Yesterday was hard. You were tired and your hip hurt, and you were worried about getting a cold. I know you were muttering a lot about hating everyone and feeling frustrated and unhelpful and dumb. It was hard. It's hard when things are hard . . . everyone feels this way sometimes. Literally anyone who was trying to write a book and manage a private practice and support their family, and also not be overwhelmed while not wanting to say no to all the requests, would feel tired and grumpy and unhelpful sometimes.

It sucks to say no to some people who want help. It does. And you are trying. And helping and trying to stay the course, right? Every no is holding space . . . for Tim and Lil and curling up at night to read and for this little book in front of you. Saying no is hard. Being imperfect is hard. And you can do this. I know you can.

I love you; I am cheering for you.

xx Kerry

Option 2b: Practise the script

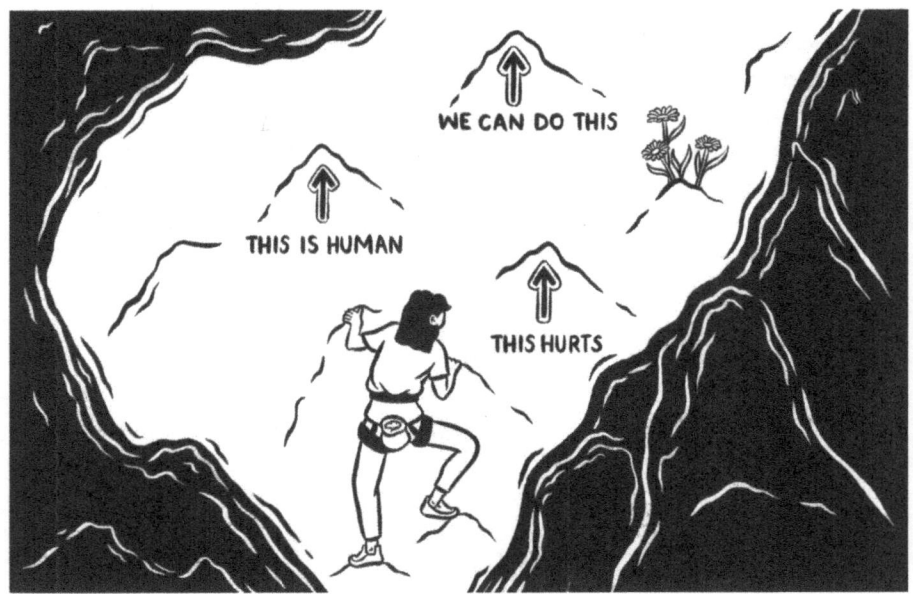

A brief self-compassion script to face challenges.

As you saw above, self-compassion can be applied in three steps.

Try the template below to develop a brief script for yourself that you can say aloud to yourself when struggles come up:

1. This is hard (add more details here, dig into what is hard).
2. This is part of being human (validate and normalise; everyone feels this way sometimes).
3. Give a kind word or encouragement to yourself (e.g. you got this; we can do this).

Kerry's examples:

» OK pause, this is hard, you're OK, slowly, slowly.
» Oh Kerry [I usually put my hand on my heart], anyone would feel this way, you are among friends.
» Wait, deep breath, you can do this, I love you.

Option 2c: Visualisation

Part of the power of self-compassion is that we soften to ourselves. Instead of beating ourselves into a better attitude, we are gently encouraging ourselves, cheering our little selves along. But many of us haven't learned to be warm and tender to ourselves. A useful alternative is to begin by accessing that gooey feeling via imagination and visualisation, then turning it to ourselves.

» Imagine a **dear friend** is having the same experience that you are. Notice any feelings of generosity, understanding and support that come up.
  - Imagine they are distressed.
  - What would you say to them?
  - How would you support them?
  - Now imagine turning that same understanding and support towards yourself.

» Imagine **yourself as a small child**. Picture a favourite outfit or a haircut from when you were small. Imagine this small child is feeling the same feelings of distress or anger or loneliness.
  - Again, notice the feelings of compassion and wanting to help arising.
  - Offer love and support to that little one, to child-you.
  - See if you can extend that same care to adult-you as well.

» Imagine you are receiving love and support from **a force larger than yourself**.
  - Some people use a favourite image from nature, a respected elder or a religious guide.
  - Notice how they accept you just as you are, expecting nothing more or less from you, offering you unconditional love and support.

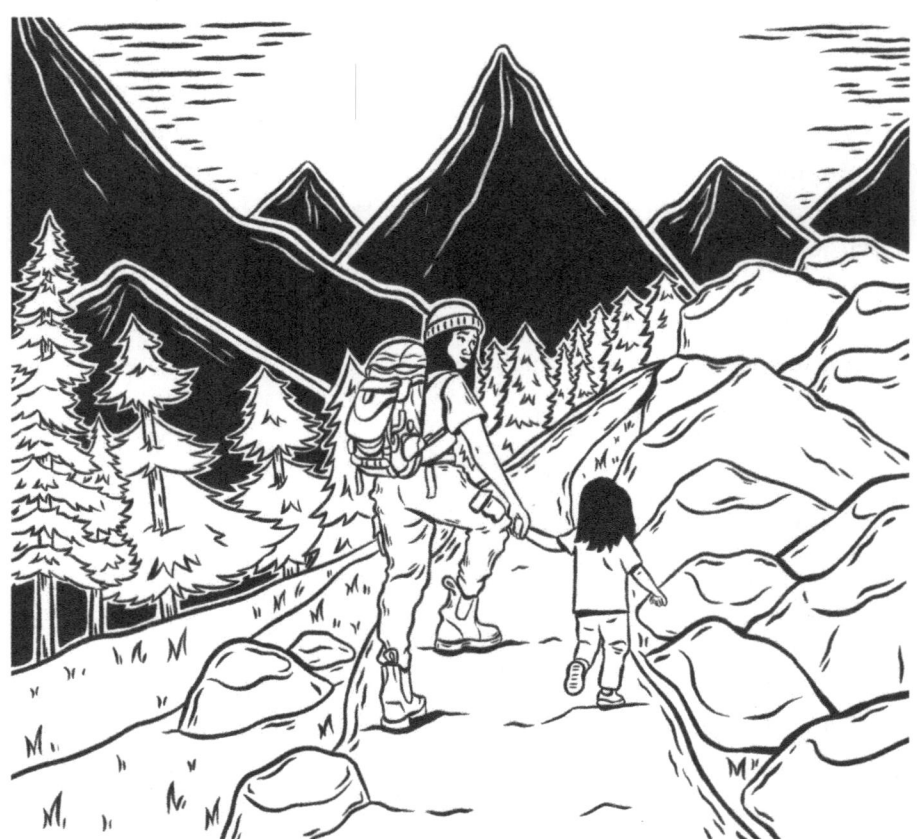

Imagine yourself as a small child. How would you speak to child-you who is having a hard time?

In my personal and professional experience, self-compassion is one of the most powerful, sustaining and wide-reaching skills that I have ever learned. Self-compassion was the life support that saved me from drowning in shame as my professional life fell apart. Manically repeating to myself, 'this is hard, anyone would feel this way, I'm cheering for you', helped me tell my mentor that I had betrayed my ethics and values because I thought I might get famous . . . or at least rich. Pressing my hand to my heart as a soothing, kind touch was the thing that empowered me to ask for help when I didn't know how to help myself. The strong kindness of self-compassion then empowered me to write a book about the experience (manically chewing three pieces of gum at a time to tolerate the terror).

Maybe the thing that continues to surprise me about self-compassion (and I'm concerned this will sound silly) is that it keeps working. I keep making different mistakes, I keep trying to learn new things and messing them up, and yet being kind to myself continues to take away the harsh edge. I guess I shouldn't be surprised, but self-compassion feels like the best vitamin boost for living. Each new step and misstep I make, as I begin to despair, the kindness trampoline bounces me back up, helping me stay on the road, try one more time, iterate and learn.

Self-compassion is the balm that helps me say to my daughter, 'I'm sorry. I'm still learning to be a mum, could I try again?' It helps me say to my clients, 'Wow, I was wrong. I apologise. Let me pause and take a breath. OK, where am I missing you? I want to do better.'

🔍 DATA

Learning and practising self-compassion makes one's life better. In a study of over a thousand people, improving self-compassion skills predicted less loneliness and higher wellbeing across five years.[ix] Writing oneself a self-compassionate letter (just like we did!) led to less depression three months later and increased happiness six months later.[x] Self-compassion promotes resilience to a myriad of life challenges,[xi] is related to less distress under stress and greater life satisfaction.[xii]

Research shows self-compassion is associated with strength, emotional and physical health, motivation, endurance and caring for others.[xiii] Across fourteen studies, people high in self-compassion experienced less anxiety, depression and stress.[xiv] I could go on and on, but I think you get the point. We practised clear seeing or accepting reality as it is. We learned to validate our experiences and struggles, being warm and kind with ourselves. Now let's transcend the details that kept us stuck and overwhelmed.

Practice 3: Perspective-taking/ metacognition

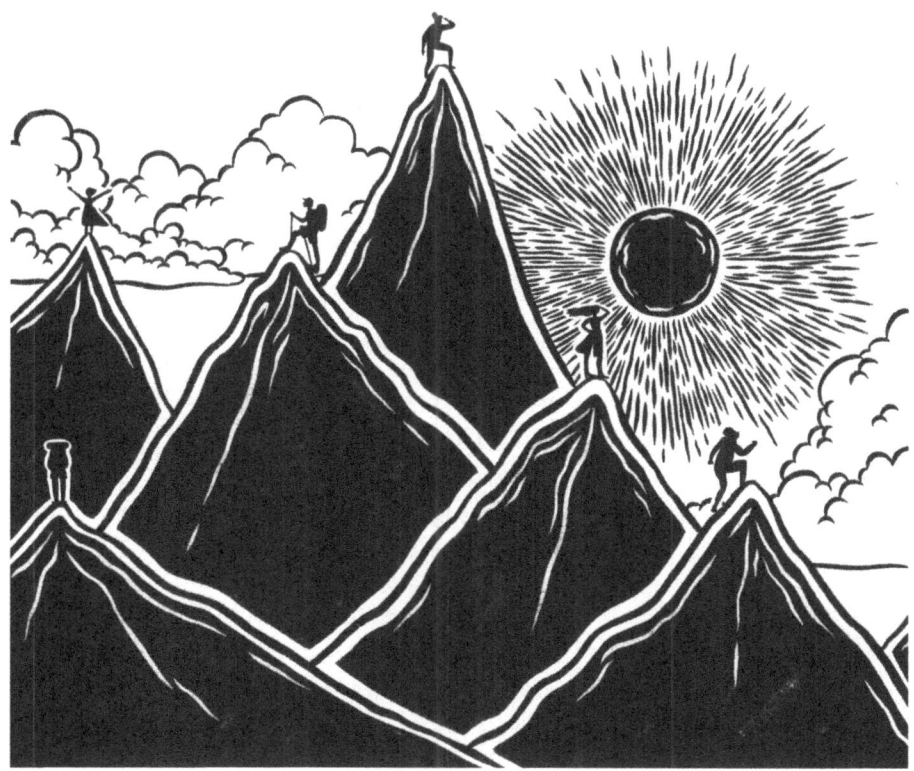

We transcend the details.

There are a few usual suspects that can lead to overwhelm:

» our expectations don't match our reality or

» our strategies to reach our goal are unworkable (and are sometimes making things worse).

For example, maybe I'm trying to be an always-available mum, and my job means performing like I have no family commitments (hmmmm, this seems unwinnable and destined for failure). In an effort to succeed in both roles, I try out some strategies that worked for short periods in the past, such as multitasking during work and family life, skipping sleep and personal care, and working longer hours. Before too long . . . overwhelm.

What if I picked up this guide instead of relying on my usual (and ineffective) coping skills of trying to do more, faster and harder?

- » Soothing would have helped me pause, breathe, and feel my exhaustion and sadness.
- » Clear seeing may have led me to recognise that this situation is fraught and unwinnable.
- » Self-compassion could have helped me unhook from guilt and shame, acknowledging my passion for both my job and my child, and settling into the knowledge that, with small adjustments, I could make things better.

At this point, you may have a clearer idea of what led to your own overwhelm.

Hopefully, you already practised showing up for yourself with kindness and compassion. Soon we will talk about concrete behaviour changes that may be helpful to relieve the overwhelm of your life. But before we can do that effectively, we must first learn to transcend the details and utilise the power of multiple perspectives.

There are many thought experiments we can use to help our minds be more flexible. I suggest three strategies, as described on the pages that follow: simplification, time travel, and heroes and mentors. Try any of these options.

You can:

- » journal about them
- » talk it out with a friend, or
- » muse while you take a walk.

Whatever works for you.

Option 3a: Simplification

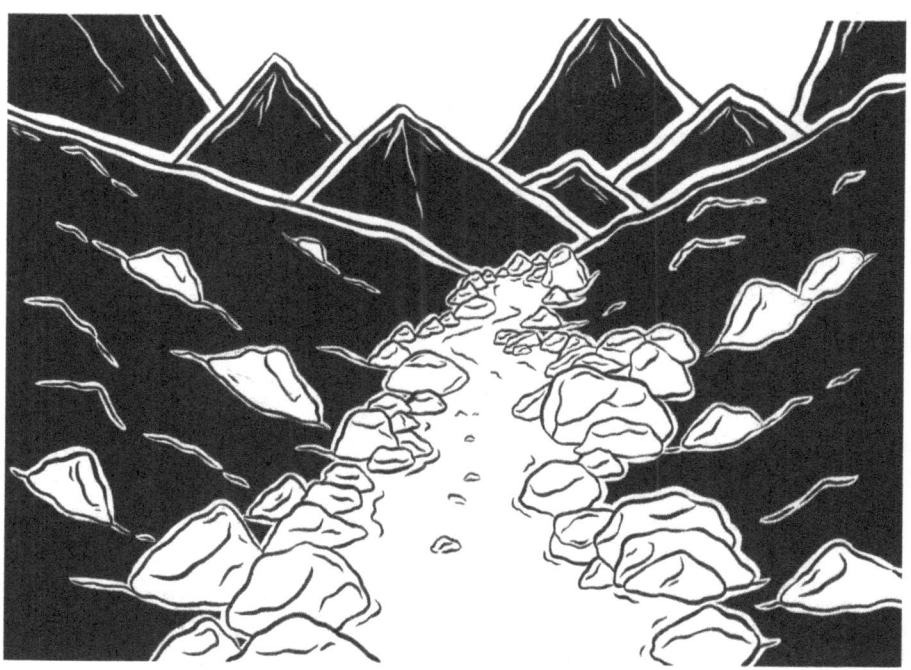

Distil the pile of details to find the essential through line.

Reflect on the following prompts, which will help you sift through the pile of details to help you find the path out and the first step forward:

- » **If I could change only one thing** about this situation, I would put all my energy into changing _____.
- » **If I was in control** of what I did, I'd do this differently:
- » **If this was easy**, I'd just . . .
- » **Urgent, important, essential and extra**
    - I know _____ feels urgent, but I'll keep remembering that _____ are the most important things to me.
    - The one essential thing I care about is _____; _____ are just distracting extras. (For example, *The one essential thing I care about is helping my partner feel loved and supported; my timeline, urgency or shoulds are just distracting extras.*)
    - My mantra for this time is _____. (Some of my favourites are 'slowly, slowly', 'flowers do not bloom in winter' and 'behind mountains are mountains'.)

Option 3b: Time travel

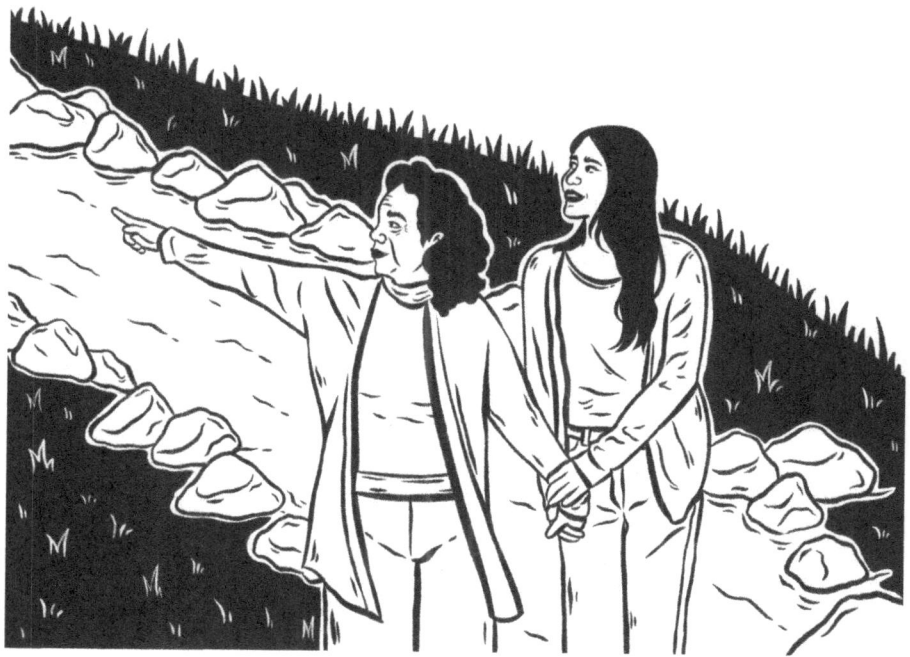

We can access great wisdom when we imagine an older, wise, compassionate future self offering us advice for now.

These prompts channel our awesome perspective-taking skills by looking backwards to a younger self or accessing our wise future self.

- » If I was giving my younger self advice about this, I would say _____.
- » If wise, balanced future me were here, they would say _____.
- » Ten years from now, the part I will still care about is _____.

Option 3c: Heroes and mentors

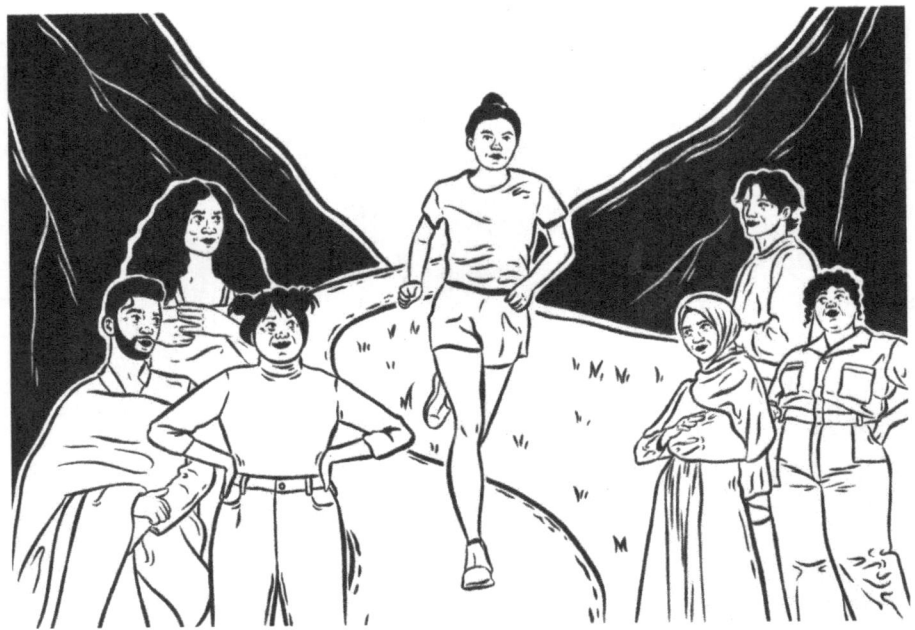

Look for answers from your historical heroes and the guides of your life.

Finally, let's reconnect in our mind with all the wisdom and inspiration we gain from others.

Practise understanding and seeing this situation from multiple perspectives:

» Pick real people who make an impact in your life (a parent, hero or mentor, sports coach, or a religious leader or icon).

» Imagine that these people are narrating your current situation. Have each of them describe what is happening.

» Imagine you are asking them for advice about your struggles.

🔍 DATA

Depending on the field of study and expertise of the researcher, perspective-taking is a skill that can fall under the broader domain of executive functioning, cognitive flexibility, behavioural flexibility or psychological flexibility.[xv] Across dozens of studies using varying and overlapping definitions of these terms, a few truths bear out:

» Flexible thoughts, behaviours and ways of relating to the world are associated with better physical health, mental health and wellbeing.[xvi]

» Rigid, inflexible thinking, behaviours and ways of relating to the world are associated with disease and lower wellbeing.[xvii]

» Interventions that increase flexibility lead to improved mental health and reduction of somatic health problems.[xviii]

Perspective-taking helps you see difficult or complex situations as 'figure-out-able', and then come up with many ideas or strategies for seeing and understanding a problem differently. As you float between different vantage points, you get new views, building a list of potential possibilities and solutions. As alluded to above, flexible thinking and acting is a skill you can build and strengthen over time, leading to cascading mental and physical benefits. Here's to perspective-taking!

Wrap-up

Last year, I wrote myself a prayer for daily use:

> *Dear Mother, please help me*
> *Accept what cannot be changed*
> *Bravely change what can be*
> *And wisely discern one from the other*
>
> *Help me live one day at a time*
> *One moment at a time*
> *Whether I understand or not*
> *Embracing this suffering world as it is*
> *Not as I wish it to be*
>
> *Help me accept hardship as a path to peace*
> *While being gentle with myself and*
> *With others, all orphans making our way home*

In a few lines, this poem suggests that we look at what is, and practise accepting the present moment, while being compassionate with ourselves and others. When we practise self-kindness, we gain the strength to look directly at our pockmarked reality. We can then accept hard truths and be empowered with new wisdom.

When we learn to transcend our old views, we are free. Now we can change what may be changed.

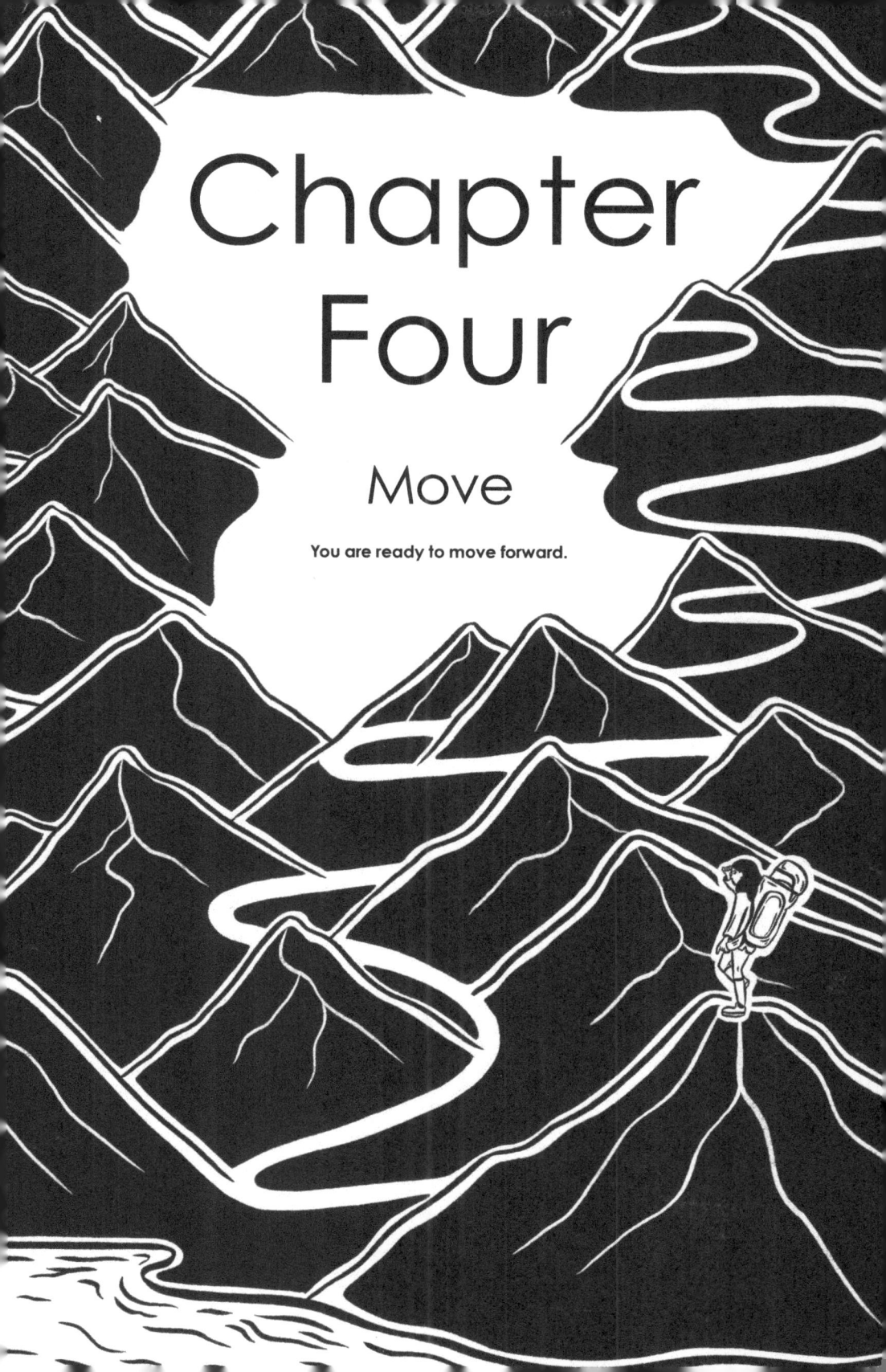

Now we understand the problems that are overwhelming us. We've looked at them clearly and tried to transcend them, practising taking multiple perspectives. With a little luck and a lot of effort, you stand here with a wider understanding of both your problems and potential solutions. With a grounded, open stance, we are ready to take action.

There is a wide array of potential 'next right steps'. Especially when life feels tight and harried, we can react quickly and without thought. My old boss used to say, 'It's all on fire, just grab a water bucket and start somewhere!'

But starting ANYWHERE can come at a great price. Starting anywhere means we are tempted to attend to the urgent at the expense of the important. I have lots of practice in this . . .

> I commit to harder, better, more
> (not slower, deeper, less)
> You know the definition of insanity?
> To do the same thing only faster
>
> – Makin-Byrd, *The Ballad of Burnout*, 2023

Instead of a scattershot path out of overwhelm, we're going to do the opposite. We will start slowly, choosing our next step with intention.

Practice 1: Set your compass

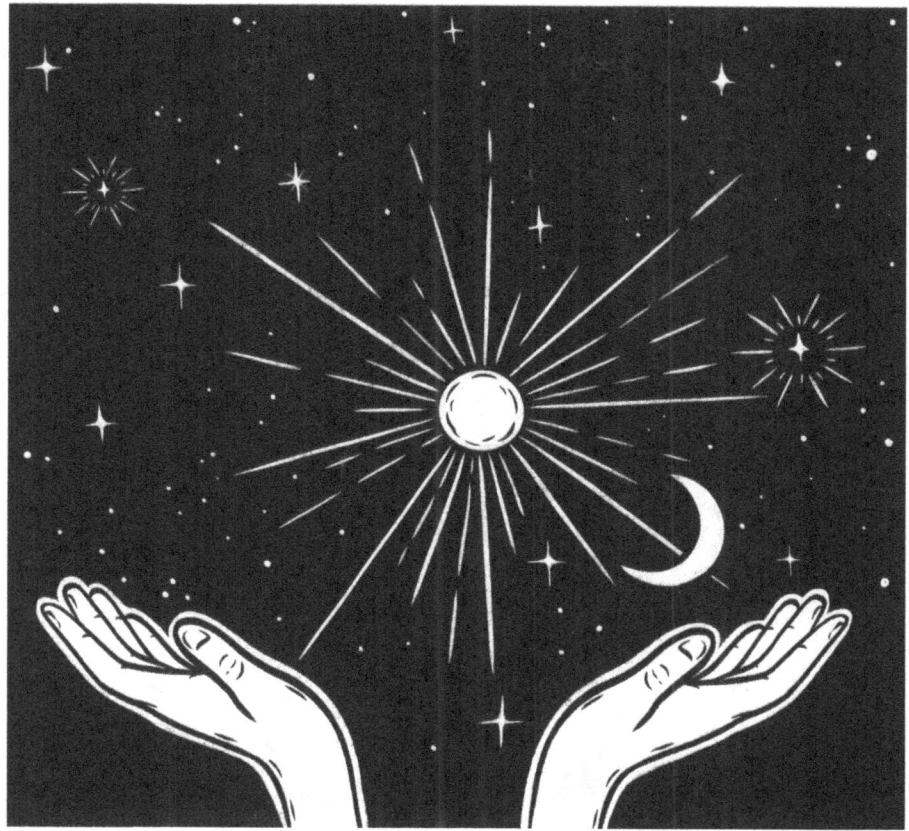

Set and check your compass regularly to keep your path true.

My friend skied across Greenland this year. Each team member took a turn leading the group. Across miles of white, barren landscape, the leader of the day would set the compass to a specific directional degree. Among the endless range of white snowfields pushing against a creamy sky, drift was inevitable, and disorientation was a realistic (and potentially fatal) concern. To keep the group safe and their path true, the compass and coordinates were checked every few minutes.

Happily, our own lives are not comprised of days of hard skiing and nights of ice camping. We aren't searching for an invisible horizon line between icy snow and a white sky. But, similarly, we can get lost among piles of requests, blindly sorting through details, trying to discern what is useful and what is distraction. For many, the tools of work and rest have coalesced into the flat expanse of a screen. We attend video meetings during the day then scroll through the night.

I'll highlight two ways that pervasive screen use can be problematic. First, we are at risk of drowning in a sea of over-information. Second, this information is available everywhere and all the time, disabling our bodies' evolved information-filtering cues of time and place.[1]

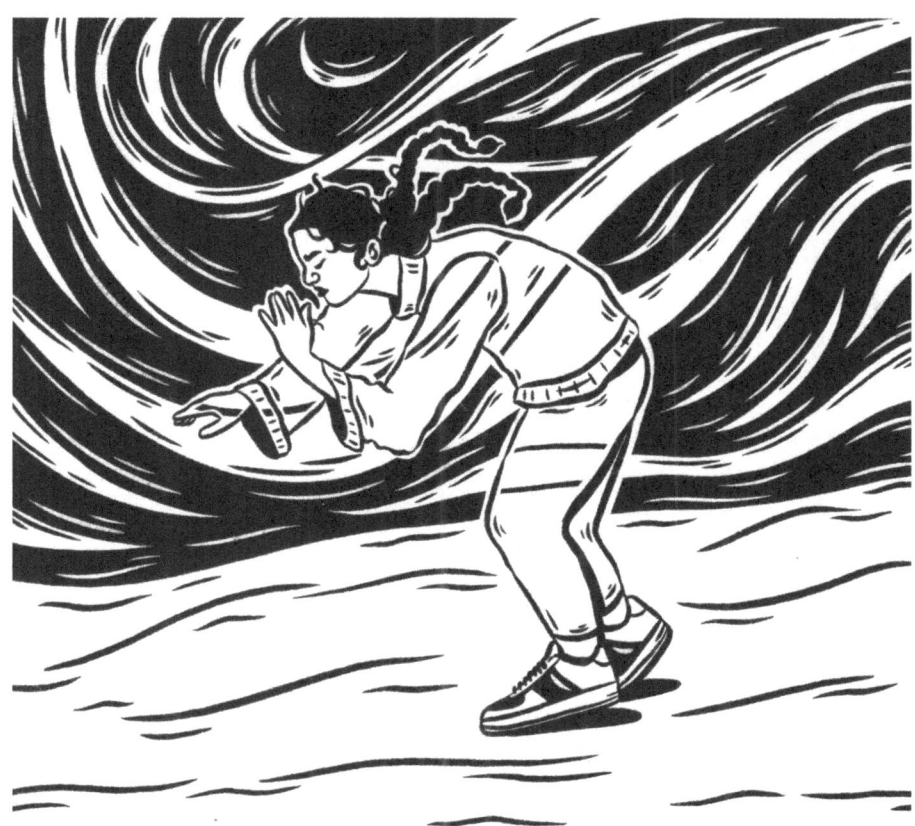

Set your compass in the over-information blizzard.

Put simply, for centuries our bodies used the cues of season, time of day and place to filter information. For example, my husband ignores the magpies in the trees most of the year. But in the spring, magpies will swoop at anyone who comes too close to their nests. So as the trees begin to bud and the weather warms, Tim changes his biking route and watches closely for magpies in his path.

Because screens collapse the normal cues of time and space, to cope we may maintain an always vigilant tension, knowing we may receive a boss's request while we're cuddled in bed with our partner, or get a mass shooting alert while reading our children their bedtime stories.

I'm here to argue that setting a compass in our over-information blizzard is just as vital as the compass needed in Greenland. A compass needle points to the Earth's magnetic north and south. Similarly, we can set our own life compass by naming and reifying the values and principles that our heart is magnetically drawn towards.

There are a variety of ways to set our compass. Each of these techniques taps into our own ideas about what we yearn for, what we most want from our lives, and where we hope to build and grow.

Option 1a: Best possible self

(First, an aside: many of the exercises in this book I have used for years in my clinical practice. Best possible self is the exception.[ii] I discovered it when researching positive psychology tools and tried it out before including it here. **It is my new favourite tip.**

Best possible self helped me be clear about what I wanted for my own new chapter of life. It helped me start doing things to build community in a new country more intentionally and deeply, without getting (as) stuck in social awkwardness, avoidance and worry.)

» In this exercise, you'll reflect on your best possible self – first by picturing it clearly, then writing about it, and finally taking a few moments to let that vision settle in your mind and heart.

» Begin by envisioning your best possible self. Research participants read this prompt: 'Imagine yourself in the future, after everything has gone as well as it possibly could. You have worked hard and succeeded at accomplishing all the goals of your life. Think of this as the realisation of your dreams, and that you have reached your full potential. Thus, you identify the best possible way that things might turn out in your life.' Just visualise this beautiful best possible life for one full minute.

» Now take fifteen minutes to write about your best possible self. Keep writing for the full time; if you get stuck, repeat what you have already written.

» After writing, take a few more minutes to imagine as vividly as possible the things you have been writing about; imagine your ideal future life in as much detail as you can.

After you complete this writing, reflect on the following questions:

» What does this tell you about what you value?

» What does it tell you about what you love and hope for in your life?

» Knowing these things, how would you like to move forward?

» What would you like to add to your life? What would you like to subtract?

Option 1b: The wonderful experience

In this writing exercise, we describe a golden moment in our life and then use it to inform our compass setting.

Research participants read this prompt: 'Think of the most wonderful experience or experiences in your life, happiest moments, ecstatic moments, moments of rapture, perhaps from being in love or from listening to music or suddenly "being hit" by a book or painting or from some great creative moment. Choose one such experience or moment. Try to imagine yourself at that moment, including all the feelings and emotions associated with the experience. Now write about the experience in as much detail as possible trying to include the feelings, thoughts and emotions that were present at the time. Please try your best to re-experience the emotions involved.'[iii]

(The quoted directions are the same instructions read by hundreds of research participants who benefited from these strategies.)

After you complete this writing, reflect on the following questions:
- » What does this memory tell you about what you value?
- » What does it tell you about what you love and hope for in your life?
- » Given this, are there any changes you would like to make to your life? Are there any ways you would like to spend your time or change your behaviour going forward?

Option 1c: Naming your values

Identify the core values that are most important to you and that you would like to guide your life.[iv]

Between the following examples and your own ideas, pick the top three values that are most important to you:

harmony   integrity   leadership   competence

peace   love   creativity   knowledge   accuracy

service   individuality   security   growth

achievement   beauty   responsibility   strength

control   consistency   truth   happiness   freedom

adventure   self-reliance

> » After you have determined your top three values (for right now), pick one value and write or reflect for a few minutes on why it is important to you.
>
> » Remember a sweet time in your life that illustrates this value.

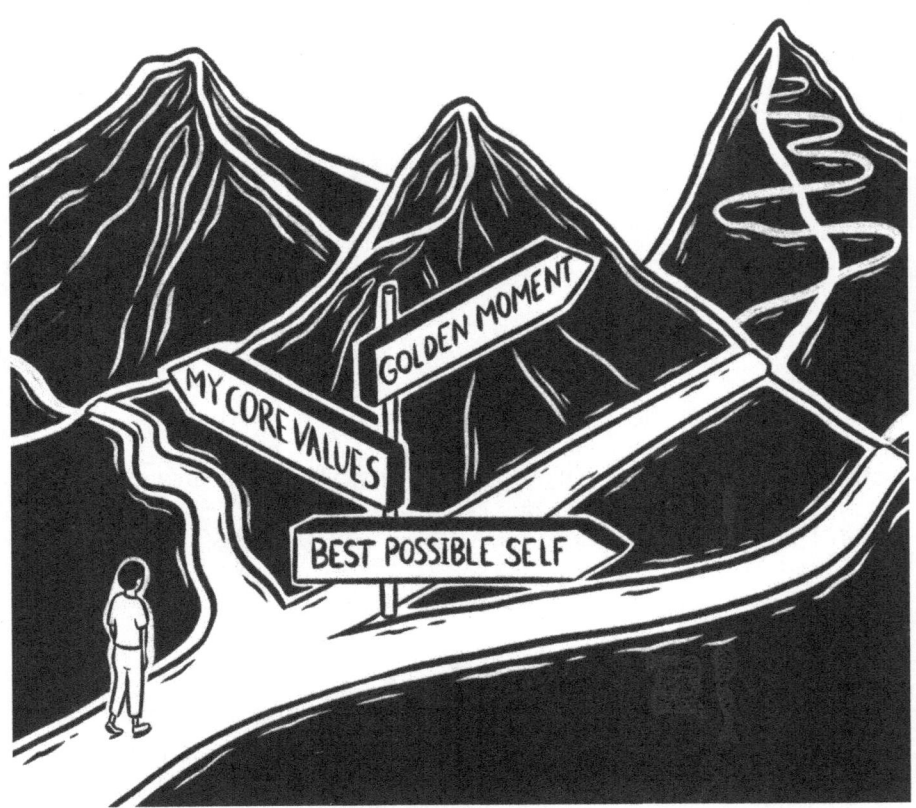

Compass-setting techniques tap into our dreams, hopes and values to suggest a blueprint for crafting our life.

🔍 DATA

The compass-setting techniques weave together a few overlapping but disparate bodies of evidence. In the early 1980s, psychologists began to examine 'subjective wellbeing',[v] or how people evaluate their lives and emotional experiences. By the early 2000s, the positive psychology movement called on psychologists to study not only mental illness but also mental health and flourishing.[vi]

Both areas of study led to robust research and the development of a number of 'brief, self-administered and cost-effective'[vii] interventions to improve wellbeing. These interventions show small but significant impacts on people's wellbeing, both immediately after completing the exercises and at three- to six-month follow-up. These effects are found both in independent randomised controlled trials and summarised in meta-analysis,[viii] the most rigorous of research evaluations.

Among a wide variety of useful positive psychology interventions, I chose to highlight the 'wonderful experience' and the 'best possible self' exercise, as they show large benefits at a small dosage. I wonder if part of what makes these interventions so powerful is their spotlight on what we most deeply care about and value.

Values are explicitly addressed in Option 3, a process also described in the literature as values clarification or values identification. This is typically the process of helping a person determine what they freely choose as personally important and yearned for.[ix] A wide variety of evidence-based techniques[x] highlight the importance of values and values-based choices. Lundgren and Larsson capture it well when they say, 'Values work can function in therapy as a motivator for change, as a metric for the effectiveness of actions, and as a guide in the development of new behavioural repertoires.'

> Or, put simply, our values point us to our heart, our wishes, our pain and our dreams, and point us home.

Practice 2: A recipe for changing your life one step at a time

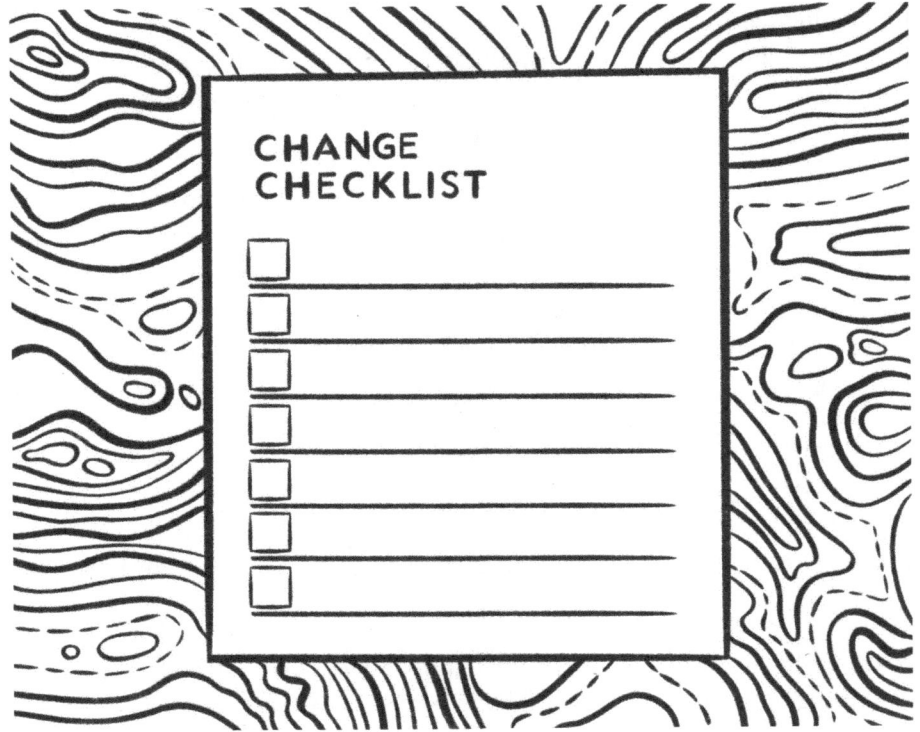

Change your behaviour and make gentle progress with these science-based steps.

We have collected a lot of information so far.

Using clear seeing, we looked at *what is*.
We practised perspective-taking to understand our struggles
from multiple vantage points.
Then we set a compass, identifying *what we wish to be*.

Now it is time to move.

Whether I like it or not, a full summary of behaviourism, evolutionary psychology, and the principles of behaviour activation and self-management are well beyond the scope of this small book and our brief time together. Instead, I've selected the key guiding principles of behaviour change that will be most useful to us now.

First, **prioritise**. After all the earlier exercises, you may have many ideas about the things you could change in your life. Just pick one or two to focus on first. We can build your whole vision over time, but for now we can begin with a single step.

Next, **define the why and how**:

» Start with your why, your purpose, your reason.

» Why are you making this change?

» Hold in your mind your wished-for goal and clearly define just one how.

» Pick one doable change you can start now, which over time will help you reach your larger goal.

Then, **optimise success**:

» Make a plan that defines a specific behaviour you can realistically accomplish with a little effort.

» Decide when and where you will do the behaviour.

» Think about ways you can celebrate your successes.

Assume there will be bumps in the road. Knowing yourself as you do, what parts will be hardest? What might get in your way? Adjust your plan to account for your predictions.

Go (and take notes). Track your progress for a few days. This doesn't need to be Darwin's field notes, just a word or two each day on what worked and what didn't.

Iterate and keep going. The perfect first plan knows it is imperfect. Channel the lessons of Darwin. Behaviour change depends on three key skills: variation, selection and retention.

» As you iterate and progress, choose what is working (selection) and keep doing that (retention).

» Make small improvements based on what you observe (variation).

» On and on, over and over, till you reach your goal.

Behaviour change form

What is true in my life now	
What I want	I value . . .
Prioritise: My first step is . . .	The biggest difference between my ideal life and my now life is . . .
	To keep growing towards my ideal life, I think I need . . .
	First steps options:
Why and how	
Optimising success: • specific realistic behaviour change • where and when • celebrating success • planning for bumps	
Go	NOTES
Integrate • continue what works, stop what doesn't • keep practising • try new variations	REVISION

Behaviour change form example

What is true in my life now	I am living in a new community and a new country. My job is pretty solitary.
What I want	I value love, connection and service. I most want to build a life full of loved ones where I'm busy with writing and providing therapy. I want to speak and write about trauma and have a busy social life with book clubs, cat volunteering and close family.
Prioritise: My first step is . . .	I am on a good track to keep doing therapy and writing. The biggest difference between my ideal life and my now life is that I don't have many local friendships and am just starting to be active in a few local clubs. To keep growing towards my ideal life, or even my goal of more connection, I think I need to keep joining clubs and meeting new people, even when I feel uncomfortable, embarrassed and shy. There really isn't a way that I can have this future ideal life without trying to make more friendships and do more out in the world. First steps options: Commit to attending one group event each fortnight (instead of cancelling at the last minute because I am avoiding awkward conversations).
Why and how	I am (barely) willing to stretch myself and feel awkward because I want to meet more friends. I want to start making relationships that could grow into my best possible vision for the future, where I feel loved and accepted and connected with more people locally. How I do this is taking small, brave steps now with strangers.

Optimising success:
- specific realistic behaviour change
- where and when
- celebrating success
- planning for bumps

- Realistic: I usually have a fortnightly invitation and am willing to dedicate that much time to doing something outside my comfort level. I commit to saying yes even if I feel worried and want to avoid it.
- I will say yes to the two book clubs, one professional group and one meditation group.
- I will write each YES on my refrigerator and buy myself a sweet treat to celebrate every two YESes.
- When I inevitably say no or have an experience that doesn't feel fun and I feel dumb, I won't just give up the whole experiment. I'll try to be kind and resilient, just taking some notes, and figure out what I could learn or do a little differently.

Go

NOTES

- Professional group: Really not fun, poorly managed and awkward. I did actually have a fun time chatting with my one friend and I met a few other people who seemed interesting.
- Book club: I was exhausted after a long week, and really didn't want to go, especially because it was only my second time, and I felt anxious about meeting new people and whether I would be as eloquent and thoughtful as they are. Went anyway (because of this stupid project), told myself it was an investment in my dream future (even though I want to just skip all the awkward beginning meetings and be one year into a comfortable book club). Really glad I went (annoyed to admit it). The whole book club was SO good, the women are really nice, and the conversation was great, begrudgingly admitting this technique apparently works.
- Meditation group: Again, felt very grumbly about this. Didn't want to drive into the city at night when I just wanted to curl up with my hubby and Lil. Did it anyway, again because of

this stupid project. Was better than I expected actually, was nice to meditate in a group. Did end up staying longer and getting to bed a lot later than I expected. So, this feels like a three out of five-star experience. One nice side-benefit was that the next week I had coffee with the meditation teacher and ended up having a really interesting conversation.

Integrate
- continue what works, stop what doesn't
- keep practising
- try new variations

REVISION

- Professional group: I'll try a few more times and make sure to carpool with my one friend I really like.

- Book club: Wow, really enjoying this. Have become more active on the text chain and am hosting next week. Feeling nervous about what they will think of our house and I want to make sure to make a nice dessert. Feeling really pleased about these relationships; two of the book club women came to my Ballad of Burnout reading. It was really nice seeing their smiling, supportive faces in the audience.

- Meditation group: Leader has been away, we moved, then I was single-parenting, so I haven't attended for about a month. I'll commit to keep attending for a few more months.

- NEW variation – exercise: Started exercising again and after a week of running had a bunch of hip pain. Started doing small runs and longer walks again. Feel like these variations are going well, definitely doing more than I would have otherwise.

🔍 DATA

The most recent advances in the field of psychology are focused on understanding the mechanisms of behaviour change.[xi]

The field is increasingly asking How do we help people change their behaviour, which changes their mood and their impact on the world around them, which over time can change their whole life?

The brief structured method proposed in this chapter is the science-based answer to this question, applied to your life. It highlighted the key nuggets from the literature on behavioural processes, contingency management, self-management, problem-solving and behavioural activation.

Note for psychotherapists interested in delving deeper: at the back of the book you'll find the main sources of inspiration in the development of my behaviour changes form.

Wrap-up

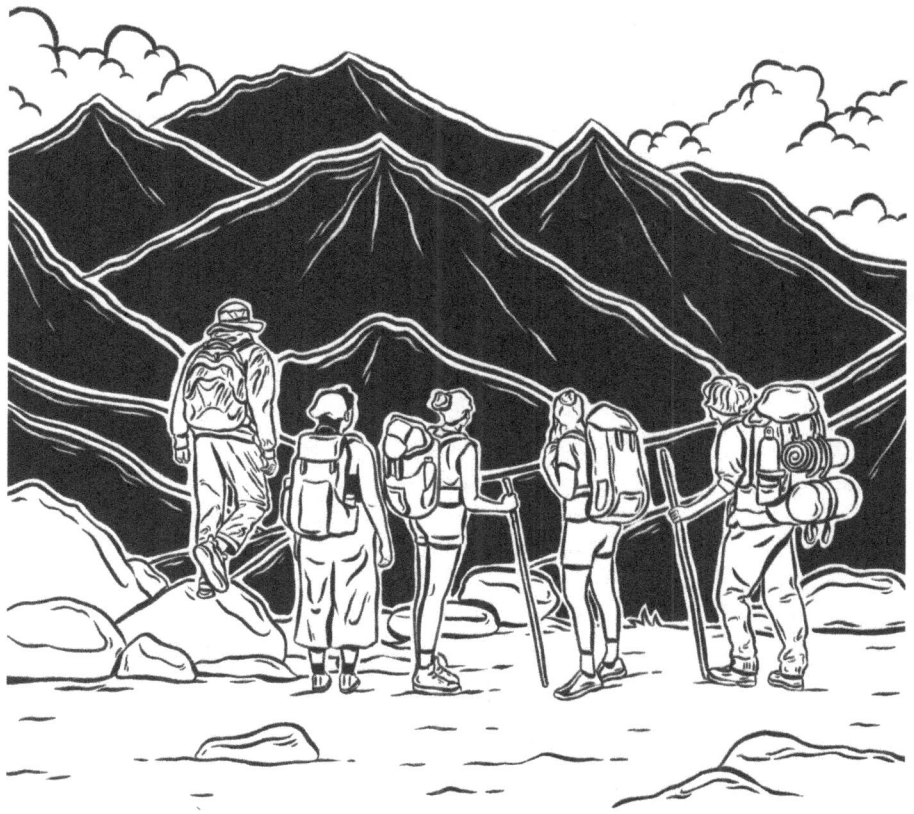

There are many paths to your version of move.

Just like there are many tracks across a vista, there are many potential paths to your personal version of 'move'. In this chapter, we focused on creating a customised plan that is rooted in what you most want and supported by a practical, smooth on-ramp. No reason to scramble up the rock face if there is a gentle switchback you could take instead.

A few weeks ago, I went to my book club even though I was tired and nervous. On the one hand, it was a trivial choice. Six out of ten times, I would have said no, gone to bed early instead, rested up and enjoyed all my convenient reasons to avoid this one commitment – there will be other book club meetings in the future, right?

On the other hand, attending book club was one small step closer to my ideal future life. To connect with my larger goals, I practised clear seeing by objectively assessing my situation. I am a new immigrant with only a few friends in the area. My last local phone call was a week earlier to an insurance salesperson. If I wanted something different, I would have to choose differently. I would have to overcome these small bumps of tiredness and nerves. **Each new stretch, each awkward conversation or night out is one more step towards my dreamed-of future – a life full of connection and local friends whom I love and am loved by.**

I hope the tools in this chapter have provided you with some ideas about how you'd like to move, what bold gentle changes you might make to get further away from overwhelm and closer to the life you are dreaming of.

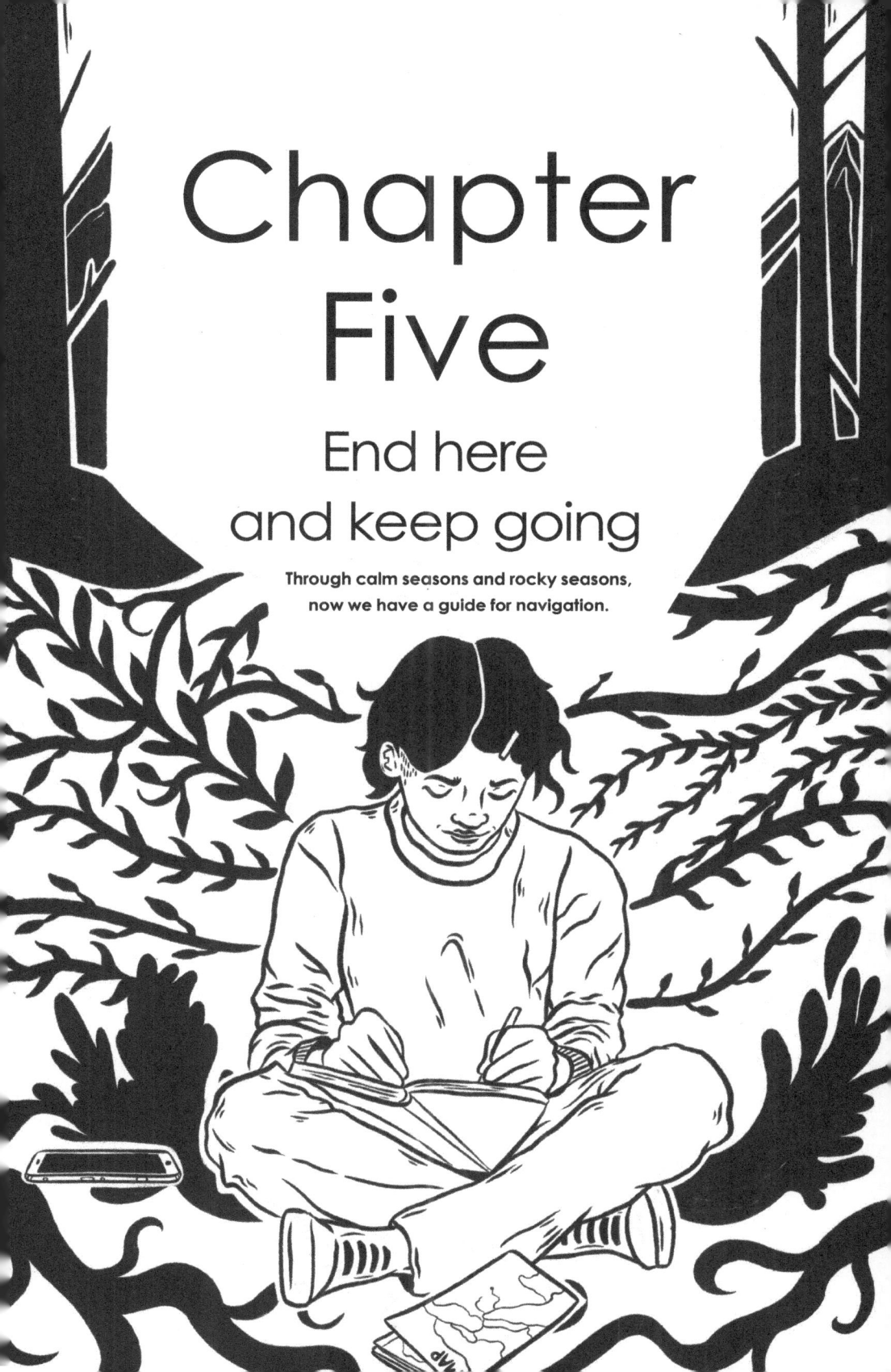

Start here

1. Soothe	*Chill out* *Breathe* *Body relaxation*
2. Transcend	*Clear seeing* *Self-compassion* *Perspective-taking/metacognition*
3. Move	*Set your compass* *A recipe for changing your life one step at a time*

5 Principles to keep going

Principle 1: Start with you

Principle 2: Continue in connection

Principle 3: Connect with the why

Principle 4: Make your world bigger

Principle 5: Let life teach you

At the beginning of this book, I told you about the times that I woke up most nights in a cold sweat. I was worried, overwhelmed and unsteady. Back then I had few local friends and a pile of meditation apps on my phone, but little idea about how to help myself sift through my stress and persistent panic. What I really needed was a brief, concrete manual to get back on my feet. And now here we are, at the almost-end of the book, having journeyed together from panic to something new.

Together, we learned to soothe our bodies when they are tight, wound up or frozen. Then we practised taking a wider lens, using clear seeing, self-compassion and metacognition to understand the life factors contributing to our overwhelm. Finally, we set a compass for a new path forward, based on our dreams and values, and we started practising gentle, meaningful change one step at a time.

What was life like for you when you started reading this book? What did you learn along the way? How are your days now?

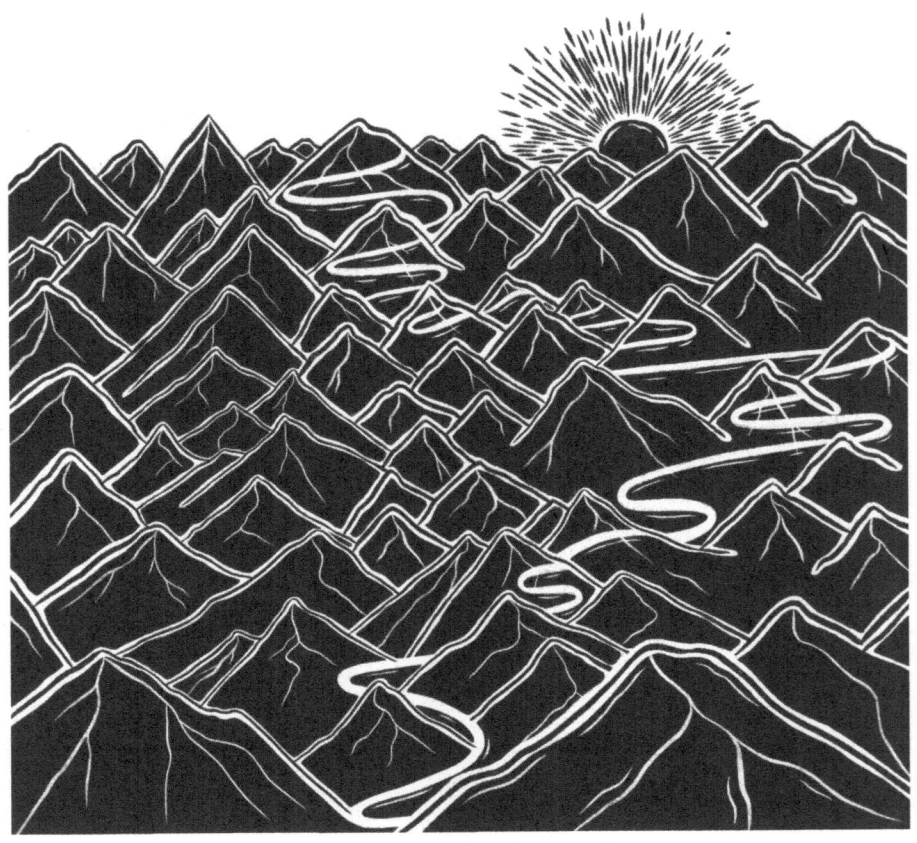

What was life like for you when you started reading this book? What did you learn along the way? How are your days now?

Just like my friend skiing across Greenland, we haven't arrived in a new perfect life, or even developed a revised super-chill personality. But we have learned some skills. Maybe we have some new perspective that we can put to immediate use as we move forward, knowing that our work will continue. We set aside our focus on a destination and embraced the journey in front of us, armed with new tools, new perspectives and new understanding.

Most of this book reviewed brief recipes and exercises to develop the skills of soothe, transcend and move. Concretely, we made small, regular changes in the minutes of our days. But over time, these small adjustments have the potential to build into momentous change. In this last chapter, let's float up one level, reviewing suggestions for practising and rebalancing across the months and years. In the following pages I propose five science-backed guiding principles to lead a life that is balanced and balancing, brimming with possibility instead of overwhelming, and sprinkled with joy to help you flourish.

Five principles for building a flourishing life

Principle 1: Start with you

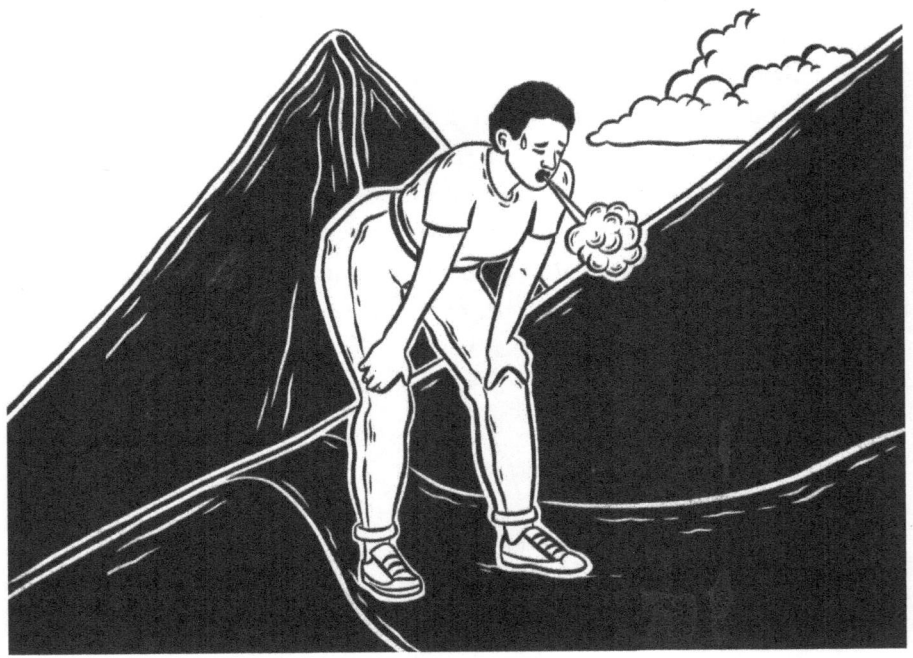

Care for yourself first, grow yourself first, give to yourself first.

When you are teetering, stretched or unsure, your first instinct may be to try to change everything, all at once. But this is actually the time to turn inwards and focus only on yourself. Set aside your grand dreams of saving the world or creating the perfect organisational system for your pantry. Care for yourself first, grow yourself first, and ask for more of yourself in order TO GIVE TO YOURSELF. When we are exhausted and stressed, our best intentions don't matter. The things we do when we are unskilful, inattentive and thoughtless can be just that – also unskilful and thoughtless. As Yongey Mingyur Rinpoche says in his book, *In Love with the World*,[1] 'Until we transform ourselves, we are like mobs of angry people screaming for peace.'

Please know that this is a lesson I (and all of us) learn, then forget, then learn again, over and over. I love the siren song of a good life hack. When I am frazzled and feel like I have control over very little, I am always tempted to charge into action. I suddenly have lots of opinions about how my husband could be working better, how my daughter could refine her sports skills and how my best friend should improve her marriage. Arrogant, thoughtless and unskilled. What I need to do is focus on my side of the street instead.

This frenzy-fuelled action is frequently also a well-masked avoidance strategy. It is harder and more pragmatic to start with ourselves, pausing and soothing, before charging forward to change the world outside ourselves. One specific day taught me this lesson. It was a Tuesday. It was the tail end of the pandemic lockdowns, and I was in the midst of my most recent burnout spiral. I hadn't seen a person outside of my family in months. My eyes were permanently sore and bleary from hundreds of hours of video meetings. Neck tight and back aching, one afternoon it was too much. I went into the backyard and lay in the grass. Just lay. (This isn't something I do . . . ever. I think this is my second time lying in the grass in about five years.) So, there I was, lying in the grass, listlessly watching leaves rustle in the breeze, admiring fantailed birds swooping from branch to branch. My daughter came home from school, walking through the back gate. I knew immediately something was wrong. Her face was still with shock, her body just beginning to shake, rippling with small earthquakes along her arms, legs and torso. She had been shouted off the road by a driver, huddling against the sidewalk as a grown man swore at her then sped away. Because I had been lazy and quiet just a second before, I came to my daughter gentle and open, not harried and tight.

What a gift those grass-lying moments turned out to be. I was the mother I wanted to be. I was tender and attentive. I can't tell you how many similar moments I've missed in the past. I literally can't tell you how many, because many times during that period she would arrive home while I was mid-meeting, or frantically responding to dozens of emails, blowing her a kiss and pointing towards her after-school snack. Sadly, probably there have been many misses. Whether we are managing unexpected crisis calls or the ordinary drone of typical tasks, starting with ourselves wins. Each moment has more potential when we show up grounded, soothed and ready.

Principle 2: Continue in connection

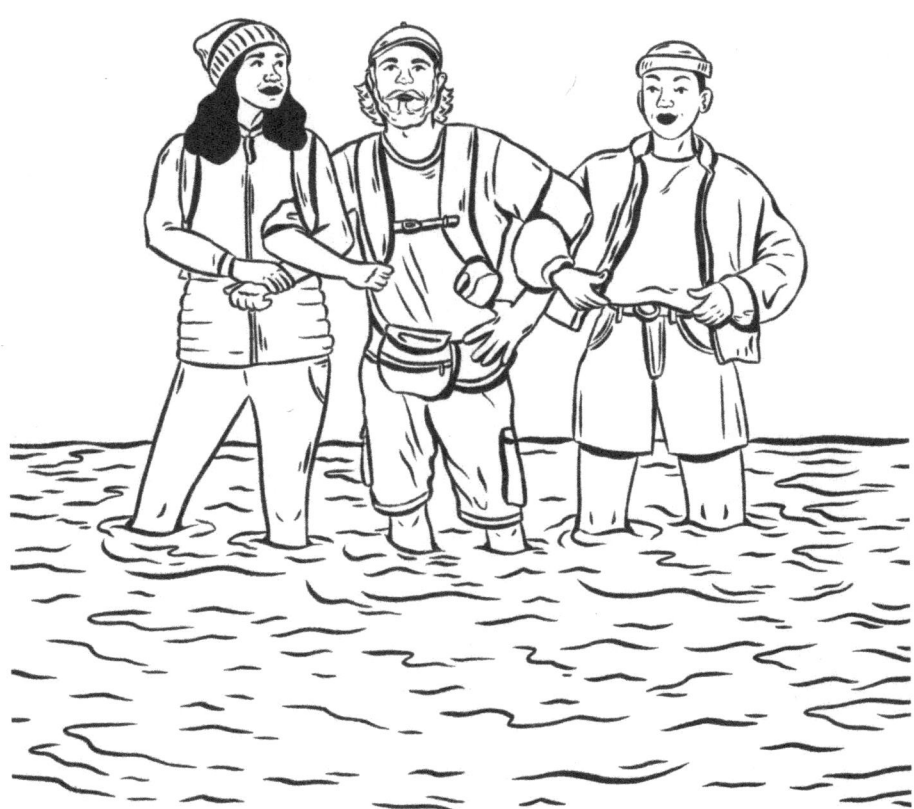

Being human is easier and more fun together.

Just as I said at the beginning of this small book, the North American and European fields of psychology and medicine have overemphasised the power and privilege of the individual for too long.[ii] As Regina Jackson and Saira Rao describe in their book *White Women*, the wellness industry has long focused on the importance of self-care and self-improvement, but this messaging can dangerously de-emphasise the impacts and healing potential of broader communities.

We evolved to be in connection. We yearn to feel belonging.[iii] Interconnection is good for us.[iv] In a world in which we are increasingly and artificially separated from others' physical presence (and from the rest of the natural world), community and belonging require attention and effort. The power of relationships can take many forms. Our connections with partners or friends, nature[v] or a presence larger than ourselves[vi] are all related to increased happiness, satisfaction, wellbeing and vitality.

Human life is a team sport; as a bonus, life is easier and more fun together. Seek or savour the communities, cultures and groups where you feel at home. For all of us, we will have moments of struggle or exhaustion across this life. We will have moments when we literally cannot go on alone. When we are already held in systems and contexts of care, we can lay back, relaxing into a larger safety net that helps and holds us.

Principle 3: Connect with the why

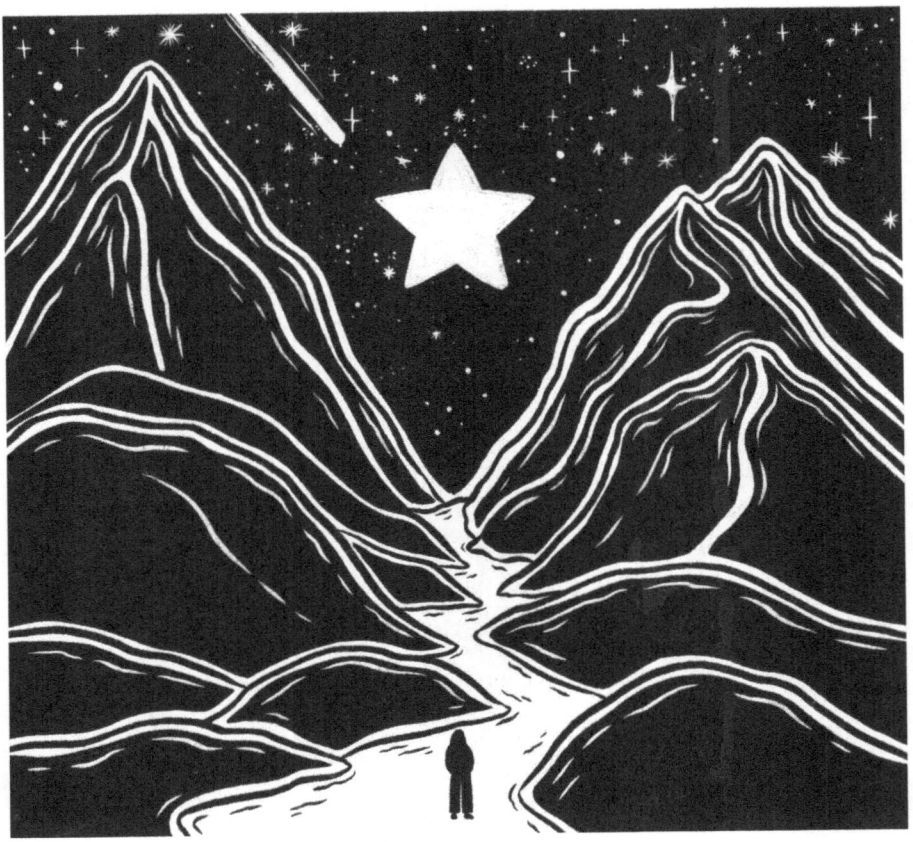

Viewing our small efforts in the context of our values and meaning gilds our work in gold.

The residents of a small village pooled their money to build a new church. A traveller wandered into the town square halfway through construction. Seeing piles of rocks and debris strewn haphazardly across a flat, dry plot of land, the traveller asked the bricklayer, 'What are you doing?' The bricklayer paused, setting down his tools to rub dust from his eyes. With a sigh he replied, 'I am laying rows of bricks, fifty long and double that wide.' The traveller nodded and wished him well. Moving deeper into the building site, the traveller came upon a lone elderly woman sweeping dust into small piles. Again, the traveller asked, 'What are you doing?' The woman leaned heavily on her broom then turned to beam at the man, 'I am building a magnificent house of worship to honour our Lord.'

As this abbreviated version of 'The Parable of the Three Bricklayers'[vii] illustrates, there are many ways to view the work we do. We can see our days as laying bricks or sending emails or washing dishes one more time. But viewing our small efforts in the context of our values and meaning gilds them in gold. We are building a cathedral, fighting for a cause, or providing hearty food and a clean home filled with love, one action at a time.

Life is hard. We grapple with big issues and our impact can feel small. When we focus on the bigness of our struggle, we can get lost easily. Instead, stay grounded in your why, in the joy of *doing* instead of the hope of an outcome. When we first moved to New Zealand, my daughter and I would comb the beaches after grand southerly storms from the Antarctic. Each post-storm shore was dotted with stranded starfish. Yes, it was the allegory that came to life. We'd walk the length of the sand, pitching the creatures back into the surf, returning them to their watery home. Just like the classic parable, we could never save them all. Yet, we saved a few. To this spiny starfish blushing orange and red, with its small active tube feet reaching wildly, to this one creature our act was the world.

When I need to be reminded of my why, I picture myself back on that beach, with one small animal in my hand. I can't help everyone. But if I can help one person, that is my reason to keep going, my own why in the world.

Principle 4: Make your world bigger

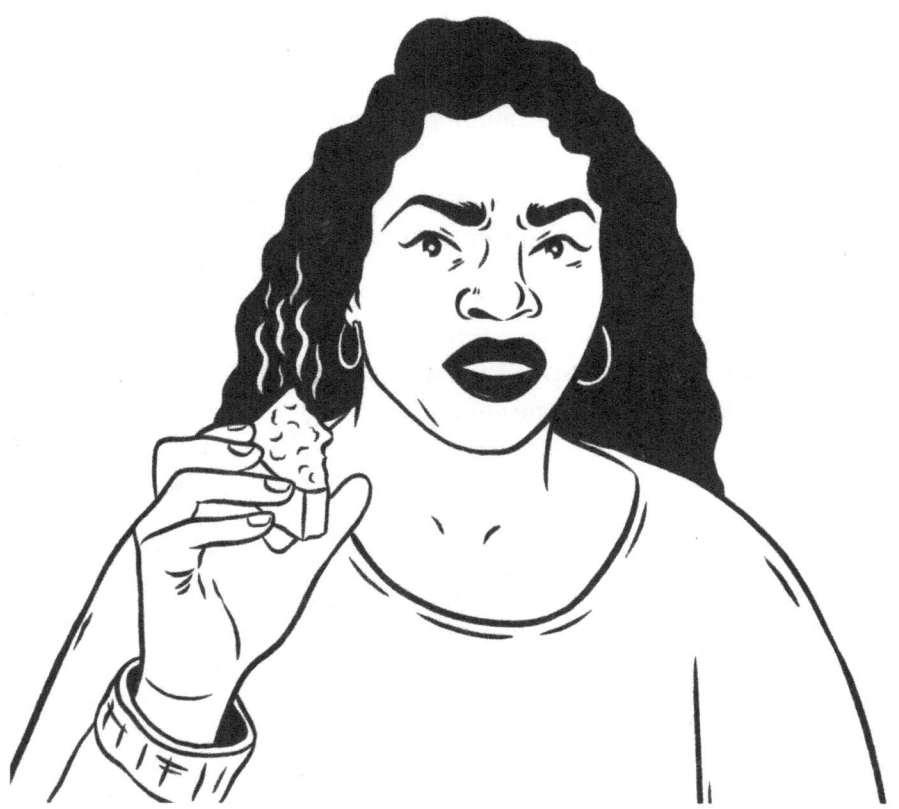

Eating stinky cheese is just one example of how small stretches can broaden our world and build our capacity.

My daughter's preschool teacher's mantra was 'Make your world bigger.' The advice worked throughout the school day:

- » During snack time: *Want a taste of pumpkin? It'll make your world bigger!*
- » During recess: *Want to see what trees look like when we stand on our heads? It'll make your world bigger!*
- » During the excitement and stress of learning about bugs: *Want to watch the bee instead of swatting at it? It'll make your world bigger.*

The advice stuck. When I wrinkled my nose at a stinky cheese or groaned at my daughter's urging to try mountain biking, she'd respond with a devilish laugh and a familiar phrase, 'It will make your world bigger.'

Humans can be a tentative species. When we experience, witness or hear about something bad happening, we learn from it. We change our behaviour to avoid distress, danger or discomfort. This can be smart, useful and good for survival.

It can also make our world smaller.

Responding to fear and anxiety with micro avoidance is pervasive in modern life. We over-limit our physical activity because of old injuries; we over-parent so we can avoid the discomfort of stepping aside and watching children experience the realities of questionable or simply uninformed decisions.

These shrinking moves cheat us (and our children) out of new learning. Our bodies can do more than we expect; our children can problem-solve and navigate much more than we predict. Without getting into a big science lecture, it serves us well to watch for small ways we may make our lives smaller over time. When you notice the pull to retreat, pause instead and look closely. Is this an intentional move or a fear-based reaction?

Awareness of our tendency to drift towards smaller and smaller is an important first step. But following that, how can we proactively try to make our world bigger? In the field of psychology, there is good evidence that experiencing positive emotions can create an 'upward spiral' of flourishing.[viii] When we practise kindness or express gratitude, we are creating a little happiness boost that makes our world bigger.

Dr Barbara Fredrickson's 'broaden and build' theory suggests that positive emotions broaden our attention, our thinking and how we relate to others. Over time, these cognitive changes build personal resources that promote health. Briefly, when we feel emotions like happiness, joy, peace or awe, we are more likely to be open and creative in our thought patterns. We are also more likely to feel trusting and connected with others. (This is true even when the positive emotion is induced or 'manipulated' by researchers in an experiment!) Over time, the cognitive and relationship benefits from positive emotions lead to a wealth of personal resources like mindfulness, mastery, positive relationships and even lower rates of illness. These personal resources in turn predict ongoing physical and psychological wellbeing.[ix]

Thus, when we savour, enjoy and induce happiness, we are investing in a self-amplifying loop that ripples out for broader and successive benefits over time.

Principle 5: Let life teach you

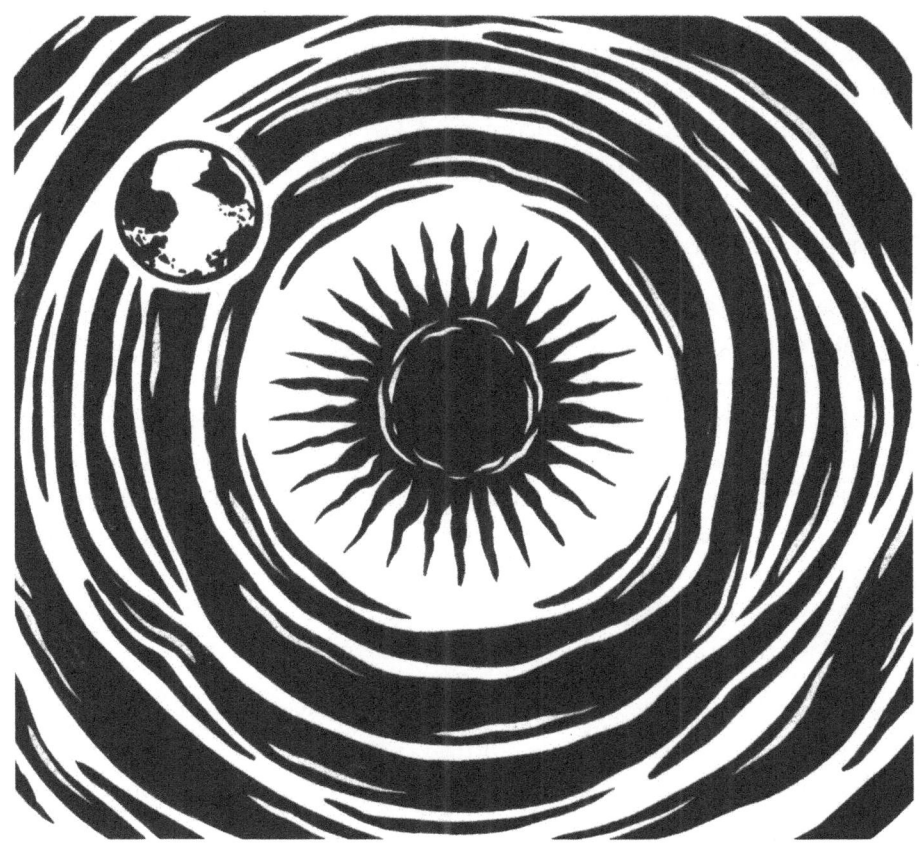

Pause and reflect at each revolution of the sun.

Finally, let life teach you. Humans aren't great at remembering things that don't align with their expectations. I know that personally I am biased towards to remembering things the way I want them to be instead of remembering reality as it is. Practically, I have found that regular reflection and journaling (or note taking) helps me track little lessons as they happen. For example, my husband and I have a long-running Google document of 'lessons learned' after each family visit. These lessons range from the mundane – *our dads like drip coffee and diet soda, buy both before they arrive!* – to the magical: *remember to ask Mum about her childhood memories of <whatever holiday is happening now>*.

I'm also a big fan of pausing at each revolution around the sun (see the 'Dr Kerry's annual review' exercise in the Appendix). Why pause each year to look backwards and plan forwards? My joints ache a bit more each year and now I look back at old photos from reunions and weddings, lingering on the faces of those people who I expected to say goodbye to soon, and also those who I am shocked are no longer here. For me, these regular reflections are useful for recognising successes, so I know what is working, and documenting my mistakes, so I can learn from them and change what isn't working. Reviewing the past year and planning for the year to come means that I make a regular date to look at where I am drifting away from the life I yearn for and reset my compass back to my true north.

It is all too easy to spend our minutes, hours and days in a haze of automatic responding. Don't just drift in a cultural current; instead, paddle heartily towards your own version of a life well lived, gently updating your course with each new learning.

The end, and a parting gift

Here is the beginning again, as we arrive at the end. You know that you can overcome overwhelm in three steps: soothe, transcend and move. You have practised and are ready to keep moving. As a parting gift, here is my favourite daily exercise:

» I notice the quick breaths, queasy stomach or harsh thoughts that signal overwhelm.

» **Soothe:** Take a few long, slow breaths, typically with my hand on my heart.

» **Transcend:** Say calmly and quietly, 'It's OK Kerry, this is hard. You can do this.'

» **Move:** Do the next right thing.

Thank you for your time, attention and energy. Thank you for trying out these exercises and for caring for your own heart, so worthy of love.

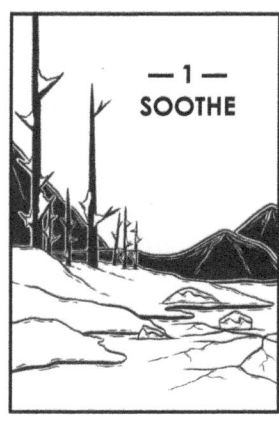 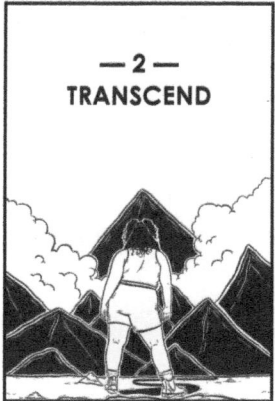 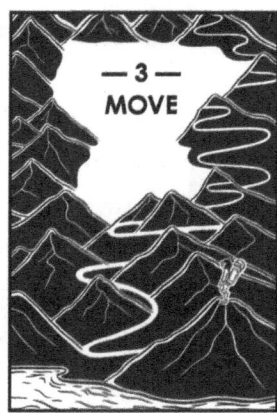

> **5 Principles to keep going**
> *Principle 1: Start with you*
> *Principle 2: Continue in connection*
> *Principle 3: Connect with the why*
> *Principle 4: Make your world bigger*
> *Principle 5: Let life teach you*

Life is hard and life is beautiful.
May we cool our heads in snowmelt streams.
May we belt out Adele and enjoy those nice long exhaled breaths.
May we see things just as they are, not as we wish them to be.

May we be kind and tender with ourselves, over and over and over.
When we are in the midst of our own (metaphorical) Greenland,
May we pause in the blinding snow
And reset our compass to our own heart.

May we change our lives just one small action at a time,
Taking notes and course correcting as we go.

May we know peace, even in a world of overwhelm.

Appendix: Dr Kerry's annual review

Looking backwards: What the last year was about

Adapt these prompts as you see fit to help you reflect on the last year (more suggestions for past year reflection can be found at drkerrymakinbyrd.com).

Last year I savoured _____
Last year I celebrated _____
Last year I struggled with _____
Last year I learned _____

Example:

Last year I focused on:	• eliminating the non-essential • finishing things I start • prioritising spending time with family.
Ways I did this:	• quit local board, resigned from community group • finished recycling project (before quitting), completed first draft of manuscript • stopped scheduling regular evening plans outside house, started doing city adventures with family, doing monthly family day.
Things I learned:	• Part of the barrier to doing less is that I feel anxious, lazy and unproductive when I do less. • I can be perfectionist and hypercritical. Building small habits accrues to significant change across a year. • It's important for me to keep practising something new through the initial discomfort phase.

Looking forwards: What this year will be about/ what I will be about

This is your mood board or inspiration for what you'd like the next year to be about (more on this at drkerrymakinbyrd.com). What would you like to feel and evoke?

What quotes or images will inspire you this year?

Example:
___

Cal Newport's writing on doing just a few things within a seasonal pace.

Jenny Odell's writing about being enough and taking pleasure in the time and space we are in.

Remember the Zach Bryan song about gratitude for today.

My guiding words for this coming year: ease and enough.

Next year's annual goals

Now let's get into concrete planning. Make a list of goals or dreams you hope to achieve. Make sure to also give yourself credit for what is going well now; your goals can (should?) include maintaining what is working and the habits you want to continue.

Some people find it helpful to organise these goals into buckets such as self, love/family, community and trade/profession. Some people have additional buckets for service, religion, fitness and making the world better.

What would you like to accomplish or practise next year?

- **SELF (this can include mental and physical health and spiritual goals)** ____
- **LOVE/FAMILY** ____
- **COMMUNITY** ____
- **TRADE/PROFESSION** ____

Example:

SELF	• daily meditation • maintain regular exercise • monthly prayer group
LOVE/FAMILY	• maintain weekly family dinner • quarterly camping trips
COMMUNITY	• quarterly beach clean-up • deepen local friendships • host a Thanksgiving party
TRADE/PROFESSION	• complete burnout talk • finish current manuscript • start next manuscript • start new training • maintain weekly newsletter

Q1 quarterly goals

Prioritise what you will do first among all your annual plans.

Pick one to three things you will focus on in quarter 1.

What would you like to accomplish or practise next year?

- SELF _____
- LOVE/FAMILY _____
- COMMUNITY _____
- TRADE/PROFESSION _____

Example:

SELF	- daily meditation - maintain regular exercise
LOVE/FAMILY	- maintain weekly family dinner - plan first camping trip
COMMUNITY	- plan one beach clean-up - plan a few dates with local friends (application of deepening local friendships)
TRADE/PROFESSION	- finish current manuscript - maintain weekly newsletter

Q1 weekly goals

Quarter 1 is simply a pile of weeks. Each week we reorient ourselves to our north stars: what this year is about and what goals we are working towards.

Some people find it helpful to match their journaling calendar segments to a work or school schedule (e.g. the financial year or the academic year). In weekly journaling, we also take notes to keep learning.

The perfect first plan knows it is imperfect. *Channel the lessons of Darwin. Behaviour change depends on three key skills: variation, selection and retention.*

- Before the week starts, set weekly goals linked to your quarterly goals.
- At the end of the week, take notes then look at what you learned.
- Moving forward, choose what is working (selection) and keep doing that (retention).
- Make small improvements based on what you observe (variation).
- On and on, over and over, till you reach your goal.

At the end of each quarter, we pause to re-evaluate and tune up our plans.

Personal note: For my own tracking, I match my quarterly and weekly tracking to the New Zealand school terms. I find it helpful for my internal planning to parallel the school year, as the school calendar necessarily dictates parts of my schedule and responsibilities. Plus, each term is ten weeks, which is a solid sprint distance to achieve concrete, measurable goals.

Q1 EXAMPLE	Guiding principles: ease and enough; do fewer things			
Q1 Goals	Daily meditation. Regular exercise.	Maintain weekly family dinner. Plan first camping trip.	Plan one beach clean-up. Plan a few dates with local friends.	Finish current manuscript. Keep regular peer group consultation meeting.
	Self	**Love/Family**	**Community**	**Trade**
Week 1 goals – did this last Friday	Meditate four out of seven days. Exercise four out of seven days.	Do one family dinner on Wednesday. Plan camping trip next week.	Skip till next week.	Do one hour of writing each weekday. Peer consult group meets next week.
Week 1 notes – completed review this Friday (end of week)	Made sense to do either meditation or exercise each day, was easier to just switch back and forth, doing one of these when I woke up each morning.	Family dinner was good, helpful to have it on everyone's calendar before the week was filled up with other plans.	Don't really want to do beach clean-up; seems like a great idea in concept but not realistic.	Couldn't always get an hour done, but committing to doing something each day was helpful; will adjust my goal to forty-five minutes daily to see if that's doable.
Week 1 revisions	Switch back and forth between exercise and meditation.	Schedule family dinner in advance. Plan camping trip next week.	Plan a few dates with local friends.	Update goal to forty-five minutes of daily writing.

Q1 weekly journals (copy more as needed)

Q1	Guiding principles:			
	Self	Love/Family	Community	Trade
Week 1 goals				
Week 1 notes				
Week 1 revisions				

Q1	Guiding principles:			
	Self	Love/Family	Community	Trade
Week 1 goals				
Week 1 notes				
Week 1 revisions				

Q1	Guiding principles:			
	Self	Love/Family	Community	Trade
Week 1 goals				
Week 1 notes				
Week 1 revisions				

Q1 quarterly journals (copy more as needed)

	Guiding principles:			
	Self	Love/Family	Community	Trade
2025 goals				
Q1 goals				
Q1 achievements				
Q1 disappointments				
Q1 learnings				
Plan for Q2				

Acknowledgements

This journal was developed with inspiration from the following resources:

- Cal Newport's thoughts on time management and his time block planner (find more information on his website or YouTube channel)
- Year compass, yearcompass.com
- Key nuggets from psychology research on behavioural processes, contingency management, self-management, problem-solving and behavioural activation, as summarised in Hayes, S. C. & Hofmann, S. G. (eds) (2018) Process-based CBT: The science and core clinical competencies of cognitive behavioral therapy. Context Press/New Harbinger Publications.

Acknowledgements

Thank you to my ancestors, to the miners and farmers and mothers and fathers and pastors and soldiers and immigrants. You worked hard and valued education and scrimped money and parented with love so I could write quietly in a room for hundreds of hours to make this book.

Thank you to my grandmother who wrote poems in her craft room and to my mother who filled journals of notes and stories. Thank you to my cousin who is the first Makin woman to traditionally publish a book and thus showed me it was possible, even for those of us from single stoplight towns.

I am fortunate to be surrounded and supported by wise, courageous, goofy, loving friends. Ara, Arlyn, Betsy, Debbie, Meg, Sanno, Stacey and Yumi, I love you with my whole heart.

Thank you to Ben Sedley, Robyn Walser and Debbie Sorenson, who all believed in me or the manuscript enough to introduce me to potential publishers.

Thank you to Andrew McAleer, the editor at Little, Brown UK who took a chance on this little book. Andrew, you are a hero to so many science-based non-fiction dreams.

Thank you to Amanda Bernardi, literary agent feminist warrior. Your energy, skill and optimism are infectious. Let's keep fighting cruelty and oppression together with a ton of love!

Thank you to Catherine Adam at Wonderbird for design and Katharine Hall for illustrations. Your gifts made the words sing and helped increase access to everyone when they are overwhelmed. Thank you to Amanda Keats and Lynn Brown for careful copy-editing, a special beast with this many citations.

Thank you to my clients and supervisees who pay me to do work that I love. Thank you to the taxpayers of Pennsylvania, California, Colorado and New Zealand, whose contributions fund the public care that I provide (either now or in the past). My writing is possible because of this financial support.

Thank you to the authors, teachers and scientists who gave their wisdom generously and are cited here.

Thank you to my extended family. Your love, practical childcare, emotional support and financial support made this book possible. Thank you to the Makins, the Byrds, the Makin-Byrds, the Hiltons and the Johnstones. Thank you to my husband and my daughter.

To Liliana and Ellie Sage, we'll keep fighting to make a better world for you.

Endnotes

Chapter 1

i   Abdalla, M., Abdalla, M., Abdalla, S., Saad, M., Jones, D. S. & Podolsky, S. H. (2023) The under-representation and stagnation of female, Black, and Hispanic authorship in the *Journal of the American Medical Association* and the *New England Journal of Medicine*. *Journal of Racial and Ethnic Health Disparities, 10*(2), 920–929.

ii   Jagsi, R., Guancial, E. A., Worobey, C. C., Henault, L. E., Chang, Y., Starr, R., Tarbell, N. J. & Hylek, E. M. (2006) The 'gender gap' in authorship of academic medical literature – a 35-year perspective. *New England Journal of Medicine, 355*(3), 281–287.

iii   Wilkerson, I. (2020) *Caste: The origins of our discontents*. Random House.

iv   Roberts, S. O., Bareket-Shavit, C., Dollins, F. A., Goldie, P. D. & Mortenson, E. (2020) Racial inequality in psychological research: Trends of the past and recommendations for the future. *Perspectives on Psychological Science, 15*(6), 1295–1309.

v   Ricard, J. A., Parker, T. C., Dhamala, E., Kwasa, J., Allsop, A. & Holmes, A. J. (2023) Confronting racially exclusionary practices in the acquisition and analyses of neuroimaging data. *Nature Neuroscience, 26*(1), 4–11.

vi   The influences of a variety of macroenvironmental or nation-level factors on subjective wellbeing summarised by Diener, E., Heintzelman, S. J., Kushlev, K., Tay, L., Wirtz, D., Lutes, L. D. & Oishi, S. (2017) Findings all psychologists should know from the new science on subjective well-being. *Canadian Psychology/psychologie canadienne, 58*(2), 87.

vii   Settles, I. H., Warner, L. R., Buchanan, N. T. & Jones, M. K. (2020) Understanding psychology's resistance to intersectionality theory using a framework of epistemic exclusion and invisibility. *Journal of Social Issues, 76*(4), 796–813.

Chapter 2

i   Porges, S. W. (2022) Polyvagal theory: A science of safety. *Frontiers in Integrative Neuroscience, 16*, 27.

ii McKay, M. (2018) Arousal reduction. In S. C. Hayes & S. G. Hofmann (eds), *Process-based CBT: The science and core clinical competencies of cognitive behavioral therapy.* Context Press/New Harbinger Publications, p. 245.

iii Don't blame me! Ackerman and colleagues demonstrated that full-body immersion has a larger impact than just getting your face wet and cold. Ackermann, S. P., Raab, M., Backschat, S., Smith, D. J. C., Javelle, F. & Laborde, S. (2022) The diving response and cardiac vagal activity: A systematic review and meta-analysis. *Psychophysiology*, e14183.

iv Placement on the right lateral neck area is intended to cool the vagus nerve. Jungmann, M., Vencatachellum, S., Van Ryckeghem, D. & Vögele, C. (2018) Effects of cold stimulation on cardiac-vagal activation in healthy participants: Randomized controlled trial. *JMIR Formative Research*, 2(2), e10257.

v Godek, D. & Freeman, A. M. (2022) Physiology, diving reflex. *StatPearls* [internet], last update 26 September. StatPearls Publishing.

vi Baranova, T., Podyacheva, E., Zemlyanukhina, T., Berlov, D., Danilova, M., Glotov, O. & Glotov, A. (2022) Vascular reactions of the diving reflex in men and women carrying different ADRA1A genotypes. *International Journal of Molecular Sciences*, 23(16), 9433.

vii Espersen, K., Frandsen, H., Lorentzen, T., Kanstrup, I. L. & Christensen, N. J. (2002) The human spleen as an erythrocyte reservoir in diving-related interventions. *Journal of Applied Physiology: Respiratory, Environmental and Exercise Physiology*, 92(5), 2071–2079. https://doi.org/10.1152/japplphysiol.00055.2001.

viii Kyriakoulis, P., Kyrios, M., Nardi, A. E., Freire, R. C. & Schier, M. (2021) The implications of the diving response in reducing panic symptoms. *Frontiers in Psychiatry*, 12, 784884.

ix Richer, R., Zenkner, J., Küderle, A., Rohleder, N. & Eskofier, B. M. (2022) Vagus activation by cold face test reduces acute psychosocial stress responses. *Scientific Reports*, 12(1), 19270.

x Tipton, C. M. (2014) The history of 'exercise is medicine' in ancient civilizations. *Advances in Physiology Education*, 38(2), 109–117.

xi Van Diest, I., Verstappen, K., Aubert, A. E., Widjaja, D., Vansteenwegen, D. & Vlemincx, E. (2014) Inhalation/exhalation ratio modulates the effect of slow breathing on heart rate variability and relaxation. *Applied Psychophysiology and Biofeedback, 39,* 171–180.

xii Cappo, B. M. & Holmes, D. S. (1984) The utility of prolonged respiratory exhalation for reducing physiological and psychological arousal in non-threatening and threatening situations. *Journal of Psychosomatic Research, 28*(4), 265–273.

xiii Hopper, S. I., Murray, S. L., Ferrara, L. R. & Singleton, J. K. (2019) Effectiveness of diaphragmatic breathing for reducing physiological and psychological stress in adults: A quantitative systematic review. *JBI Database of Systematic Reviews and Implementation Reports, 17*(9), 1855–1876.

xiv Busch, V., Magerl, W., Kern, U., Haas, J., Hajak, G. & Eichhammer, P. (2012) The effect of deep and slow breathing on pain perception, autonomic activity, and mood processing – an experimental study. *Pain Medicine, 13*(2), 215–228.

xv Balban, M. Y., Neri, E., Kogon, M. M., Weed, L., Nouriani, B., Jo, B., Holl, G., Zeitzer, J. M., Spiegel, D. & Huberman, A. D. (2023) Brief structured respiration practices enhance mood and reduce physiological arousal. *Cell Reports Medicine, 4*(1), 100895.

xvi Tensing for longer may be even more effective! O'Bannon, R. M., Richard, H. C. & Runcie, D. (1987) Progressive relaxation as a function of procedural variations and anxiety level. *International Journal of Psychophysiology, 5*(3), 207–214.

xvii Script adapted from McKay, M. (2018) Arousal reduction. In S. C. Hayes & S. G. Hofmann (eds), *Process-based CBT: The science and core clinical competencies of cognitive behavioral therapy.* Context Press/New Harbinger Publications, p. 245.

xviii Schultz, J. H. & Luthe, W. (1959) *Autogenic training: A psychophysiologic approach to psychotherapy.* Grune & Stratton.

xix First came You must relax, by Jacobson, E. (Whittlesey House, 1934), then a standardised protocol for empirical research was published: Bernstein, D. A. & Borkovec, T. D. (1973) *Progressive relaxation training: A manual for the helping professions.* Research Press.

xx Manzoni, G. M., Pagnini, F., Castelnuovo, G. & Molinari, E. (2008) Relaxation training for anxiety: A ten-years systematic review with meta-analysis. *BMC Psychiatry, 8*, article 41. https://doi.org/10.1186/1471-244X-8-41.

Stetter, F. & Kupper, S. (2002) Autogenic training: A meta-analysis of clinical outcome studies. *Applied Psychophysiology and Biofeedback, 27*, 45–98.

xxi   Chellew, K., Evans, P., Fornes-Vives, J., Perez, G. & Garcia-Banda, G. (2015) The effect of progressive muscle relaxation on daily cortisol secretion. *Stress, 18*(5), 538–544.

xxii   Agee, J. D., Danoff-Burg, S. & Grant, C. A. (2009) Comparing brief stress management courses in a community sample: Mindfulness skills and progressive muscle relaxation. *Explore, 5*(2), 104–109.

xxiii   Rausch, S. M., Gramling, S. E. & Auerbach, S. M. (2006) Effects of a single session of large-group meditation and progressive muscle relaxation training on stress reduction, reactivity, and recovery. *International Journal of Stress Management, 13*(3), 273.

Chapter 3

i   RAIN: The nourishing art of mindful inquiry. Tricycle Online Courses: https://learn.tricycle.org/p/rain

ii   RAIN: Recognize, allow, investigate, nurture. Tara Brach resources: www.tarabrach.com/rain

iii   Anheyer, D., Haller, H., Barth, J., Lauche, R., Dobos, G. & Cramer, H. (2017) Mindfulness-based stress reduction for treating low back pain: A systematic review and meta-analysis. *Annals of Internal Medicine, 166*(11), 799–807.

iv   Creswell, J. D. (2017) Mindfulness interventions. Annual Review of Psychology, 68, 491–516.

Hofmann, S. G., Sawyer, A. T., Witt, A. A. & Oh, D. (2010) The effect of mindfulness-based therapy on anxiety and depression: A meta-analytic review. *Journal of Consulting and Clinical Psychology, 78*(2), 169.

Keng, S. L., Smoski, M. J. & Robins, C. J. (2011) Effects of mindfulness on psychological health: A review of empirical studies. *Clinical Psychology Review, 31*(6), 1041–1056.

v   Hayes, S. C., Strosahl, K. D. & Wilson, K. G. (2012) *Acceptance and commitment therapy: The process and practice of mindful change* (2nd edn). Guilford Press.

vi   Hayes, S. C., Villatte, M., Levin, M. & Hildebrandt, M. (2011) Open, aware, and active: Contextual approaches as an emerging trend in the behavioral and cognitive therapies. *Annual Review of Clinical Psychology, 7*, 141–168.

vii   As summarised by Neff, K. D. (2023) Self-compassion: Theory, method, research, and intervention. *Annual Review of Psychology, 74*, 193–217.

viii   This exercise is adapted from the work of Dr Kristin Neff and the teachings of Dr Kelly McGonigal.

ix   Lee, E. E., Govind, T., Ramsey, M., Wu, T. C., Daly, R., Liu, J., Tu, X. M., Paulus, M.P., Thomas, M. L. & Jeste, D. V. (2021) Compassion toward others and self-compassion predict mental and physical well-being: A 5-year longitudinal study of 1090 community-dwelling adults across the lifespan. *Translational Psychiatry, 11*(1), 397.

x   Shapira, L. B. & Mongrain, M. (2010) The benefits of self-compassion and optimism exercises for individuals vulnerable to depression. *Journal of Positive Psychology, 5*(5), 377–389.

xi   As summarised by Neff, K. D. (2023) Self-compassion: Theory, method, research, and intervention. *Annual Review of Psychology, 74*, 193–217.

xii   Babenko, O., Mosewich, A. D., Lee, A. & Koppula, S. (2019) Association of physicians' self-compassion with work engagement, exhaustion, and professional life satisfaction. *Medical Sciences, 7*(2), 29.
McDonald, M. A., Meckes, S. J. & Lancaster, C. L. (2021) Compassion for oneself and others protects the mental health of first responders. *Mindfulness, 12*, 659–671.
Weng, H. Y., Lapate, R. C., Stodola, D. E., Rogers, G. M. & Davidson, R. J. (2018) Visual attention to suffering after compassion training is associated with decreased amygdala responses. *Frontiers in Psychology, 9*, 771.

xiii   Neff, K. D. (2023) Self-compassion: Theory, method, research, and intervention. *Annual Review of Psychology, 74*, 193–217.

xiv MacBeth, A. & Gumley, A. (2012) Exploring compassion: A meta-analysis of the association between self-compassion and psychopathology. *Clinical Psychology Review, 32*(6), 545–552.

xv Doorley, J. D., Goodman, F. R., Kelso, K. C. & Kashdan, T. B. (2020) Psychological flexibility: What we know, what we do not know, and what we think we know. *Social and Personality Psychology Compass, 14*(12), 1–11.
Ionescu, T. (2012) Exploring the nature of cognitive flexibility. *New Ideas in Psychology, 30*(2), 190–200.
Kashdan, T. B. & Rottenberg, J. (2010) Psychological flexibility as a fundamental aspect of health. *Clinical Psychology Review, 30*(7), 865–878.
Uddin, L. Q. (2021) Cognitive and behavioural flexibility: Neural mechanisms and clinical considerations. *Nature Reviews Neuroscience, 22*(3), 167–179.

xvi Howell, A. J. & Demuynck, K. M. (2021) Psychological flexibility and psychological inflexibility are independently associated with both hedonic and eudaimonic well-being. Journal of Contextual Behavioral Science, 20, 163–171.

xvii Kashdan, B. & Rottenberg, J. (2010) Psychological flexibility as a fundamental aspect of health. *Clinical Psychology Review, 30*(7), 865–878.

xviii A-tjak, J. G., Davis, M. L., Morina, N., Powers, M. B., Smits, J. A. & Emmelkamp, P. M. (2015) A meta-analysis of the efficacy of acceptance and commitment therapy for clinically relevant mental and physical health problems. *Psychotherapy and Psychosomatics, 84*(1), 30–36.
Bai, Z., Luo, S., Zhang, L., Wu, S. & Chi, I. (2020) Acceptance and commitment therapy (ACT) to reduce depression: A systematic review and meta-analysis. *Journal of Affective Disorders, 260*, 728–737.

Chapter 4

i Odell, J. (2024) *Saving time: Discovering a life beyond productivity culture.* Random House Trade Paperbacks.

ii Peters, M. L., Flink, I. K., Boersma, K. & Linton, S. J. (2010) Manipulating optimism: Can imagining a best possible self be used to increase positive future expectancies? *Journal of Positive Psychology, 5*(3), 204–211.

iii	Burton, C. M. & King, L. A. (2004) The health benefits of writing about intensely positive experiences. *Journal of Research in Personality, 38*(2), 150–163.
iv	Wagner, C. C. & Sanchez, F. P. (2002) The role of values in motivational interviewing. *Motivational Interviewing: Preparing People for Change, 2*, 284–298. Supplemented from values derived from Enneagram types: www.enneagraminstitute.com/type-descriptions.
v	Diener, E. (1984) Subjective well-being. *Psychological Bulletin, 95*(3), 542.
vi	Seligman, M. E. & Csikszentmihalyi, M. (2000) *Positive psychology: An introduction* (Vol. 55, No. 1, p. 5). American Psychological Association.
vii	Diener, E., Heintzelman, S. J., Kushlev, K., Tay, L., Wirtz, D., Lutes, L. D. & Oishi, S. (2017) Findings all psychologists should know from the new science on subjective well-being. *Canadian Psychology/psychologie canadienne, 58*(2), 87.
viii	As summarised by Bolier, L., Haverman, M., Westerhof, G. J., Riper, H., Smit, F. & Bohlmeijer, E. (2013) Positive psychology interventions: A meta-analysis of randomized controlled studies. *BMC Public Health, 13*(1), 1–20.
ix	Lundgren, T. & Larsson, A. (2018) Values choice and clarification. In S. C. Hayes & S. G. Hofmann (eds), *Process-based CBT: The science and core clinical competencies of cognitive behavioral therapy*. Context Press/New Harbinger Publications, pp. 375–388.
x	Such as acceptance and commitment therapy, behavioural activation and motivational interviewing.
xi	Hayes, S. C. & Hofmann, S. G. (eds) (2018) *Process-based CBT: The science and core clinical competencies of cognitive behavioral therapy*. Context Press/New Harbinger Publications.

Chapter 5

i	Rinpoche, Y. M. & Tworkov, H. (2021) *In love with the world: A monk's journey through the bardos of living and dying*. Random House Trade Paperbacks.
ii	Jackson, R. and Rao, S. (2022) *White women: Everything you already know about your own racism and how to do better*. Penguin Random House.

iii   Leary, M. R. & Baumeister, R. F. (1995) The need to belong. *Psychological Bulletin, 117*(3), 497–529.

iv   Fiske, S. T. (2018) Social beings: *Core motives in social psychology.* John Wiley & Sons.

v   Capaldi, C. A., Dopko, R. L. & Zelenski, J. M. (2014) The relationship between nature connectedness and happiness: A meta-analysis. *Frontiers in Psychology, 5*, article 976.

vi   Rizvi, M. A. K. & Hossain, M. Z. (2017) Relationship between religious belief and happiness: A systematic literature review. *Journal of Religion & Health, 56*(5), 1561–1582. https://doi.org/10.1007/s10943-016-0332-6.

vii   This is my own adaptation of 'The Parable of the Three Bricklayers', originally published in *What can a man believe?*, a 1927 book by Bruce Barton.

viii   Garland, E. L., Fredrickson, B., Kring, A. M., Johnson, D. P., Meyer, P. S. & Penn, D. L. (2010) Upward spirals of positive emotions counter downward spirals of negativity: Insights from the broaden-and-build theory and affective neuroscience on the treatment of emotion dysfunctions and deficits in psychopathology. *Clinical Psychology Review, 30*(7), 849–864.

ix   Fredrickson, B. L. (2004) The broaden-and-build theory of positive emotions. *Philosophical Transactions of the Royal Society of London. Series B: Biological Sciences, 359*(1449), 1367–1377.

Behaviour change form references

What is true in my life now	- Problem definition from contemporary problem-solving therapy (Nezu, Greenfield & Nezu, 2016)
What I want	- Externalisation and visualisation from contemporary problem-solving therapy (Nezu, Greenfield & Nezu, 2016)
Prioritise: My first step is . . .	- SSTA – or stop, slow down, think and act – from contemporary problem-solving therapy (Nezu, Greenfield & Nezu, 2016) - Pick a single behavioural target from contingency management (Higgins, Silverman & Washio, 2011); similar to simplification from contemporary problem-solving therapy (Nezu, Greenfield & Nezu, 2016) - Define a target behaviour and behavioural goal from self-management (Sarafino, 2011; Watson & Tharp, 2014)
Why and how	- Link your behavioural goal to your outcome goal from self-management (Sarafino, 2011; Watson & Tharp, 2014) - Values and reinforcement from behavioural activation (extensive work summarised in Martell, 2018) - Values choice and clarification from bull's eye values survey as summarised by Lundgren & Larsson (2018) - Values in ACT as summarised by Luoma, Hayes & Walser (2007) - Values card sort and discussion from motivational interviewing (Miller & Rollick, 2002, 2013

Optimising success: – specific realistic behaviour change – where and when – celebrating success – planning for bumps	• Define the objective clearly from contingency management (Higgins, Silverman & Washio, 2011), self-management (Sarafino, 2011; Watson & Tharp, 2014) and motivational interviewing (Miller & Rollick, 2002, 2013) • Managing operant antecedents from self-management (Sarafino, 2011; Watson & Tharp, 2014) • Choosing positive reinforcers from self-management (Sarafino, 2011; Watson & Tharp, 2014) and from motivational interviewing (Miller & Rollick, 2002, 2013) • Activity structuring and scheduling from behavioural activation (extensive work summarised in Martell, 2018) • Identifying barriers from behavioural activation (extensive work summarised in Martell, 2018) and motivational interviewing (Miller & Rollick, 2002, 2013) • Developing a change plan from motivational interviewing (Miller & Rollick, 2002, 2013)
Go (and take notes)	• Monitor progress frequently from contingency management (Higgins, Silverman & Washio, 2011) • Collecting data on implementation from self-management (Sarafino, 2011; Watson & Tharp, 2014; although I bet these authors would recommend we collect baseline data before starting to make changes) • Solution implementation from contemporary problem-solving therapy (Nezu, Greenfield & Nezu, 2016) • Activity monitoring from behavioural activation (extensive work summarised in Martell, 2018)

Integrate – continue what works, stop what doesn't – keep practising – try new variations	• Solution verification from contemporary problem-solving therapy (Nezu, Greenfield & Nezu, 2016) • Taken together, the recommended process uses the principles of modern evolution science: variation, selection, extinction and retention. We try new things (variation), selecting actions that we expect may bring us closer to our valued goals, then evaluate how this is working. We retain that which is successful and useful, stop what isn't, and keep iterating new ideas (variation again). Optimally, this variation is customised and flexible to context.

Subscribe to the OVERCOMING NEWSLETTER for health practitioners

Sign up here to our quarterly email for health practitioners and mental health workers:
overcoming.co.uk/7/#signup

This will keep you up to date about the latest publications, news, free resources and blog posts from the Overcoming book series and other self-help publishing. You can also find other book content and free downloadable resources at www.overcoming.co.uk and follow us on Twitter @overcominglb

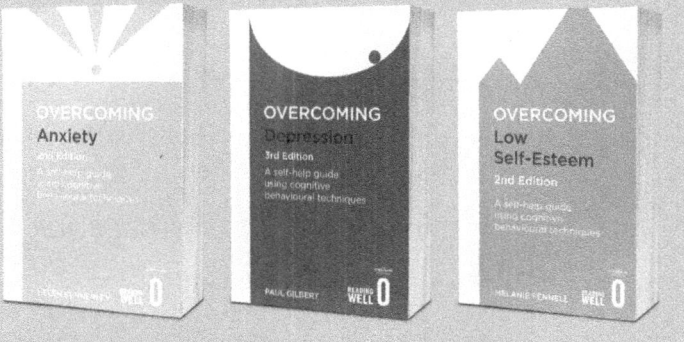

Holding the Heavy Stuff:
Making Space for Critical Thoughts and Painful Emotions
Ben Sedley

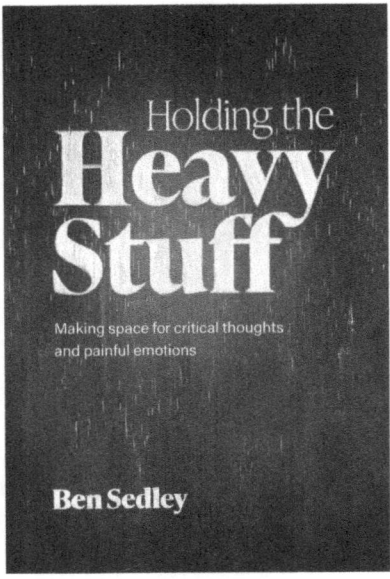

Holding the Heavy Stuff **is a unique, illustrated self-help guide for anyone who has struggled with low mood, worries, self-doubts or mean thoughts about themselves and then found it difficult to move their life forward.**

It is for people who feel overwhelmed or consumed by worries about the future, or find themselves stuck reliving moments from their past.

It is for those who have days, weeks or months when sadness takes over and getting through each hour feels challenging.

It is for those who can't imagine life getting better as the world gets worse.

It is for people who feel dumped on or knocked off track.

It is for all of us who face tragedy and difficulty and feel weighed down.

Perhaps you struggle to live the life you want or are holding too much heavy stuff. The more you try to fight this internal pain, the more you have it. Instead of struggling against it, this book offers a different approach. You will learn ways to carry the heavy stuff with you as you go where you want to go.